PRAISE FOR *PUSH*

"Technology today gives us the ability to shape training around the uniqueness of every individual—their body, their dreams, their aspirations. When exercise speaks this personal language, it delivers results that inspire, and those results ignite the deepest motivation. Dr. Jordan D. Metzl's *Push* captures this spirit, reminding us that movement is not only science—it is the poetry of health and longevity."

—Nerio Alessandri, CEO and founder of Technogym

"Motivation is the bridge between medical advice and measurable outcomes. When patients find a reason to move, exercise becomes the most reliable prescription we have—extending healthspan, preserving muscle, and quieting the inflammation that fuels chronic disease. In *Push,* Dr. Metzl shows us that medicine works best when our patients move. Motivation turns 'I should' into daily action—and those small, consistent pushes add years to life and life to years."

—Bryan Kelly, MD, MBA, president and CEO of HSS,
Surgeon-in-Chief Emeritus, Chief Emeritus of the Sports Medicine
Institute, and the Ellen Wright Chair in Musculoskeletal Research

"*Push* is overflowing with Dr. Metzl's boundless enthusiasm for movement. He is one of the rare physicians who lives in the worlds of both fitness and medicine. His goal: Healthy longevity for all."

—Robert Sallis, MD, former president of American College of
Sports Medicine and team physician of Los Angeles Clippers
and Los Angeles Football Club

"I have watched Dr. Metzl build a fitness community of thousands where he teaches others to embrace their fitness motivation. *Push* is a must-read for those who are looking to find their own 'get up and go' personal consult with Dr. Metzl."

—Daphne Scott, MD, service chief of Primary Sports Medicine
and former orthopedic and sports medicine consultant of UFC

"The critical importance of motivation is summed up well by the famous Nelson Mandela who said, 'Do not judge me by my successes, judge me by how many times I fell down and got back up again.' *Push* makes clear the incredible importance of motivation for individuals to start and then maintain a personal fitness program. This book explores the scientific underpinnings for motivation, providing key insights to help keep you motivated to pursue a healthy lifestyle!"

—Scott Rodeo, MD, head team physician of New York Giants Football and prior head team physician of U.S. Olympic Swimming Team

"Jordan Metzl has inspired and strategically encouraged us to transcend the boundaries we once believed limited our physical capabilities. In *Push,* he masterfully uncovers the hidden elements that drive our exercise and physical activities, delving into the essential emotional and mental components that define our performance. This book is not just an exploration, it's a revelation that empowers readers to redefine what they can achieve!"

—Karen Sutton, MD, team physician of U.S. Ski & Snowboard and team physician of USA Lacrosse

PUSH

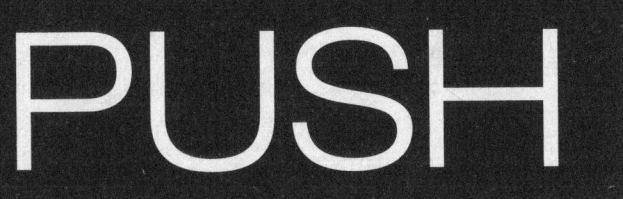

PUSH

UNLOCK THE SCIENCE OF FITNESS MOTIVATION TO EMBRACE HEALTH AND LONGEVITY

Jordan D. Metzl, MD

with Mike Zimmerman

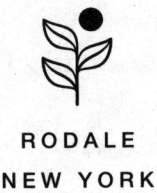

RODALE

NEW YORK

Rodale Books
An imprint of Random House
A division of Penguin Random House LLC
1745 Broadway, New York, NY 10019
rodalebooks.com | randomhousebooks.com
penguinrandomhouse.com

A Rodale Trade Paperback Original

Library of Congress Cataloging-in-Publication Data
Names: Metzl, Jordan D., author | Zimmerman, Mike author
Title: PUSH / Jordan D. Metzl, Mike Zimmerman.
Description: New York, NY: Rodale, [2026] | Includes bibliographical references.
Identifiers: LCCN 2025028738 (print) | LCCN 2025028739 (ebook) |
ISBN 9781623365882 trade paperback | ISBN 9781623365899 ebook
Subjects: LCSH: Exercise | Motivation (Psychology) | Physical fitness
Classification: LCC RA781 .M4467 2026 (print) | LCC RA781 (ebook)
LC record available at https://lccn.loc.gov/2025028738
LC ebook record available at https://lccn.loc.gov/2025028739

Printed in the United States of America

1st Printing

BOOK TEAM: Production editor: Robert Siek • Managing editor: Allison Fox •
Production manager: Richard Elman • Proofreaders: Robin Slutzky and Ying Gao

Book design by Mary A. Wirth
Exercise illustrations by Kagan McLeod

First Paperback Edition

The authorized representative in the EU for product safety and compliance is
Penguin Random House Ireland, Morrison Chambers, 32 Nassau Street,
Dublin D02 YH68, Ireland. https://eu-contact.penguin.ie

*This book is dedicated to the blessed memory
of my dear father, Dr. Kurt Metzl, who taught me
how to push myself in mind and body.*

*This knowledge not only helped me succeed but taught me
how to push my patients and community to succeed as well.
Victories I have achieved are due in large part to his relentless
perseverance and all-encompassing support.*

You must be the change you wish to see in the world.

—MAHATMA GANDHI

Commit to getting off your ass.

—JORDAN D. METZL, MD

CONTENTS

PART THREE

The Push Plan

99

PART FOUR

Build Your Own Workouts

163

Movement: A Love Story

Alice, a college professor, has been coming to me for years. When she was in her late sixties, she experienced a two-year span where she lost her husband, received a breast cancer diagnosis, and fell into a deep depression, during which she had to simultaneously mourn her partner and her life as she knew it.

Of course, we all know that as our age creeps forward and years pile up, life tends to take more than it gives. But this was almost too much. As she later told me, "I just didn't know what the point of life was anymore."

When living reaches the point of pointlessness, there's not a lot you can say to that person. "It'll all be okay." Yeah, no. Call it whatever you want, the end of the line, rock bottom, Alice had reached that point of pointlessness. So, you know what she did?

She went for a walk, which turned into a slow run.

This smart, accomplished woman who had been hollowed out by loss and disease tied her sneakers and went out the door.

She didn't pull a Forrest Gump and run to the opposite ocean and back. But after her run that day—which in truth wasn't all that long— she went out and did it again the next day. She ran and she kept running to fight her disease, aid her recovery, and stare down her sadness.

After some months, she entered a race. And another race after that. Then, at age seventy, with her cancer and depression in remission, she ran her first marathon. After that, she ran another marathon. As of this writing, Alice has run fifteen marathons.

She comes to me with the classic aging endurance athlete issues, usually achy knees. But we also talk. Over the years, I've gotten her started on a strength-training program to prevent losing muscle (heck, she *increased* it) and protect her bone density. So now she's a fully engaged, wildly independent, seriously motivated eighty-something who runs 26.2 miles and teaches a kettlebell class. Now *she's* motivating people.

But that first day—that first run. Why did she do that?

Why?

On my first day of medical school, in the first lecture, the logic of becoming a doctor was explained to me the same way it's explained in medical schools around the world. The practice of medicine, from the time of Hippocrates in ancient Greece up to today, tells us to always ask the first and most important question: Why? This question, so simple and yet so incredibly important, is the basis of medicine. Why did the patient spontaneously lose consciousness, why does her shoulder hurt, why is he having headaches? Without first wondering why, we can never search for an answer. Sometimes the answer is obvious and sometimes hidden. But we must always ask.

Why?

When it comes to motivation, the why is especially murky. When we tell patients what to do to improve their health, from undergoing routine screenings to staying away from certain vices to taking critical medications—and even then they don't do any of it—it's difficult to understand why people make unhealthy choices.

Then some patients take the opposite approach. They start a healthy behavior such as walking ten thousand steps per day, and over years they push to meet that goal. They lift weights, they swim, they dance. They become Alice. They're not dissuaded by rain or snow, they keep going, day after day, month after month, year after year.

Why?

As a sports medicine physician who is not only taking care of patients but also trying to get them to move every day to maximize their health, I have learned over time that the great white whale of compliance—sticking to a good thing no matter what—is creating healthy motivation in my patients. Why do some people commit to movement while others struggle? More important, what can I do to better understand and encourage people to embrace their own fitness motivation?

If I had the quick answer to this question, I wouldn't have had to write this book. What I've found is that fitness motivation is an incredibly complex subject. When you ask this particular "why," you can't just say "because I said so."

You have to look for clues, and what you'll learn is that each of us has our own unique set of clues big and small. This book, drawing on my own experience as a sports physician, fitness instructor, educator, and athlete, is an attempt to better understand and master the complicated world of fitness motivation.

Alice is our first clue.

Why did Alice go out for that run?

She didn't know it at the time, but it was about falling in love again.

Looking for a Great First Date

Imagine you are exactly as you are now—except for one difference. You move as much as a typical three-year-old.

How would your average day be different?

You'd park your car and run to the grocery store entrance. You'd run upstairs when it's time to bathe (or maybe you'd stomp your feet with exaggerated high-knee steps the whole way). You'd sprint to the potty because you're so lost in whatever activity you're doing you forgot you had to go.

At work you'd swing your lower legs while you sit in your chair. You'd roll your chair around your office too. You might even spin your chair around during meetings. Co-workers would race you to the coffee machine. On home-office Zoom calls you'd be the one having to mute yourself because of your literal bouncing off walls.

Sofa time in front of the TV would involve more endless leg

swinging and eventually rolling around from one end to the other (possibly even a somersault or two) and watching your favorite show while hanging your head upside down off the sofa cushion.

At bedtime, foreplay would begin with a few minutes of jumping up and down on the bed. After that, it might get really interesting.

My point: A three-year-old is in love with movement.

Most adults hate it.

52%

U.S. adults who meet the Physical Activity Guidelines for aerobic physical activity

35%

U.S. adults who meet the Physical Activity Guidelines for muscle-strengthening activity

28%

U.S adults who meet the Physical Activity Guidelines for both aerobic and muscle-strengthening activity[1]

Right there—that shift that probably begins somewhere in our teen years, that evolution from wanting to move all the time to never wanting to move *for any reason,* explains the general poor health of our society.

It explains how you feel right now.

Somewhere along the line, you fell out of love with movement.

Why? That's a complicated answer and it's in this book. But my goal is clear. *I want you to fall in love with movement again.*

My relationship with movement can be classified as a sizzling love affair. I can't quit movement. I'm Gomez, my workouts are Morticia. If I can't move, I don't feel alive.

I know I'm an outlier.

65.3 million

Number of U.S. adults considered "physically inactive"—25.3 percent of the adult population.[2] Total based on 258 million adults in the 2020 U.S. Census.

Falling back in love with movement isn't automatic. It begins with words but requires action. Most of my injured patients are passionate about getting back to regular, healthy movement again. But in almost every case where I've seen someone start moving again, I've also watched love blossom. The movement makes them happier, fitter, more vital, and more in tune with everything else in their lives.

I love that Alice found love again, especially in her golden years. She could've lived a much shorter life under a dark cloud, going with the negative motivational flow of her body and mind. "It was so easy to disengage," she says. "Retreating was the only thing that felt right to me. But feeling right didn't make it right. I knew that. If I wanted to live, I had to do the opposite of what my mind and body wanted me to."

The shoes went on her feet. Her feet took her out the door.

Talk about a great first date.

Step into My Office!

And welcome. Think of this book as a nice long consult with me. As of this moment, you stopped being alone in your journey to get healthier. Community, as you'll soon see, is one of the biggest factors in helping people embrace more positive behavior. So even if you don't literally join my IronStrength online community, you're now your very own little part of that community, and, as I said, you're not alone anymore. You can come here anytime you need a boost.

As we sit down in my office, I can already guess what you want to talk about. Why? Experience. I've been a sports doctor for twenty-five years now and an MD for more than thirty. I can say, conservatively, that I've treated more than fifty thousand patients. That's a lot of knees, backs, and shoulders. I was trained to think of them that way—*okay, here's a case of runner's knee, how do I fix it*—as body parts, or interlocking body parts when, say, knee and calf issues cause ankle and plantar issues. Anatomical puzzles to solve, and I got good at it.

I'm not the doctor I was twenty-five or even ten years ago, however. Alice, among some other memorable patients I'll tell you about, is partly responsible for my evolution as a physician. With each patient comes a story—their individual story—and I started paying attention to these stories. I slowly realized that the sore knee wasn't just a temporary ailment I could help cure. The knee (or the back or the shoulder) was a conduit into the patient's entire life. (There's a name for this now—narrative medicine—where physicians take into account all the things that make up a patient's circumstances, their medical "story.")

If I fix Alice's sore knee, she's back to training for marathons. If she's doing that, then she's also mobile and active in her social life, a full member of her community, making a positive impact on people she interacts with daily. And I realized, whoa—that one sore knee affects a lot of people. The world is literally a better place when Alice's knee doesn't hurt.

That's mind-blowing.

Think about yourself: *The world is a better place when you're healthy.* Being healthy is great for you, but also for all the people around you.

Now do the people-math on more than fifty thousand patients. That's a community the size of a small city—with each individual linked up with their own families and friends and all the people they touch.

See how this is so much bigger than just a sore knee?

Find Your Motivational Center

Add all that up and I'm no longer just a sports medicine physician. I'm a doctor, an athlete, and a fitness instructor, and all of those worlds are constantly intersecting.

I invited you to step into my office and I meant it. My office has become a motivational center as well as a healing place, a place not just to get well but to get better (so is this book!). And a while back I had an idea.

I ran my first marathon in 1998. My pledge to myself after my first marathon was to run one marathon per year. I've pretty much kept to it. Recently, I looked in an old box in my closet where I throw the race medals that are given out at the end of marathons and triathlons. The box was pretty full. And while I don't dwell on the races I finish or look back at all those miles logged, I knew this box meant something. It represented, in one tangled mess of ribbons and shiny things, all my motivation to move.

Another mind-blowing moment for me.

I needed to share that. And since I wanted my office to have that atmosphere of motivation, I took all the medals and hung them in my office under a placard that says *Always Earned, Never Given.*

I wanted to remind myself, and my patients, that the key to fitness success isn't just doing something once, it's committing to maintaining activity day after day, year after year, forever. Included in these medals are marathons from this year's New York City Marathon and from my very first in Boston, where the ribbon is frayed from years of being kept bunched up in the closet.

In each of these events and the other things I do, there's always a moment where I ask myself, "Is this really worth it?" I could be sitting on the couch watching football, but instead I'm out here pushing my body. It's not always easy. In fact, it's often hard as hell, both mentally and physically, but inside I have a voice that reminds me that it's always important to keep moving, to keep pushing ahead. Like Dory in *Finding Nemo,* "Just keep swimming."

I want to help you rediscover your own motivational voice. At first glance, this might seem to be only a beginner problem, or something for a person who hasn't been active recently or maybe ever. Nope. Even a vigorously active person will, at some point, need to fight through unhealthy motivation, and this book will help distill why and how. Example: Me! I'm always either training for some race or maintaining the fitness I already have. Doesn't seem like I would ever need to push myself for anything, but I do. In my sports medicine practice and in my own fitness life, I've taken care of many thousands of patients and run many thousands of miles. What I've noticed is if I don't push myself, over time I lose the passion for it. Even though I love movement, it gets old, it gets tough, it gets repetitive. I force myself to remember: Because of my evolution as a doctor and athlete, I am now armed with much more knowledge about the importance of consistency and intensity. Consistency, doing your exercise day after day, week after week, year after year, is the key to mental, physical, and metabolic health. And part of this equation is not only doing it but also doing it with some level of intensity. I've increasingly recognized the importance of intensity in maintaining health across your lifespan.

My passion for fitness and medicine led to the third part of my career. More than ten years ago, I started teaching fitness classes called IronStrength, focused on building and maintaining functional strength. At first, these classes were a way to keep my muscles strong with a group of like-minded people so I could continue to compete in events (and beat my brother). Over time, the entire endeavor spiraled upward and these classes became a public health initiative to promote exercise and fitness for preventive health. Our workout community morphed into one of the largest physician-led fitness initiatives, a way to get more than ten thousand people each year moving and strengthening in unison. The classes grew from twenty people in the basement of a gym to more than one thousand people on the flight deck of an aircraft carrier, and along with it, so did my passion for harnessing the motivation of a group to encourage the entire community to push ahead.

My three perspectives—sports medicine physician, athlete, and fitness instructor—have joined together to create this book, *Push*. I've written a handful of previous books, all with an aim to keep people moving, but I've never explored the nature of the mental game behind movement. Motivation felt like a logical progression for me. In my world, I tell every patient that I see, and every person who comes to my fitness classes, and every medical student and resident who comes to my office to learn, about the importance of movement for preventive health. The medicine of movement is 100 percent effective for everyone and, unlike any other drug, has no side effects. It works for everyone, young and old, rich and poor. The medicine of movement improves both lifespan (lived years) and healthspan (vitality during lived years). We are also hearing more and more about musclespan, the maintenance of muscle mass over time that affects both lifespan and healthspan. All of this ties into "inflammaging," the concept that many of the chronic diseases we see, from diabetes to heart disease to certain types of cancer, are related to a chronic inflammatory state in the body. Daily movement and maintaining healthy muscle mass lower the so-called inflammaging effect and extend our healthspan. In my world, we know all of this. But how do I get people to change their behavior? How do I get them moving day after day, month after month, year after year?

I am constantly encouraging my patients to do more. If I'm seeing you for your shoulder injury, once it's fixed, I then focus on how we can keep you moving ahead on your playing field of choice. Behind all of this is the science of motivation. What makes some people push while others don't? What do we know about the different facets of personal motivation? Is it nature? Is it nurture? What can we do to enhance our motivation, to help us all push ahead?

I wish the science of motivation was as clear as seeing a torn ligament on an MRI. We have to dig deeper. We have to push to understand ourselves.

I think it's worth it.

THE HEALTHSPAN-LIFESPAN PROBLEM
(AND SOLUTION)

Anyone who scrolls social media will eventually come across some form of the following: An influencer (with little or no medical or science background) will show the world how they've beaten the aging process and solved longevity and are spending X amount of money each month to keep their bodies at a biological age of twenty-three. Or something like that.

This book is not about that brand of "longevity." *I'm* not about that brand of longevity.

I mentioned healthspan and lifespan just now. Humanity's done a good job extending lifespan over the past one-hundred-plus years, but now we have the Healthspan-Lifespan Gap, which is the number of years between living in relatively good health and death. A 2021 *Nature* study showed average global life expectancy at about 73.2 years.[3] Meanwhile our average healthspan was 64 years, a gap of 9.2 years. The same researchers published new data in late 2024 showing the Healthspan-Lifespan Gap wider, at 9.6 years globally.[4] But in the United States? 12.4 years.

Back in 2000? 8.5 years. So the Healthspan-Lifespan Gap continues to widen. And now the U.S. Healthspan-Lifespan Gap amounts to more than 15 percent of our lives spent in deteriorating health. That's a long time.

Spoiler alert: Regular exercise can extend healthspan and help close the gap. We want our healthspans and lifespans to be as close as possible.

Here's what I mean: I recently saw a patient who is ninety-one years old. He's in good health, and I don't believe it's any coincidence that he bikes four times a week, strength-trains three times a week, and walks three times a week. He came to see me about some hip pain and wanted to be sure he could keep moving as he healed. He's all better now—and still moving.

I can't say how much longer this man will live, but when his time is finally up, his Healthspan-Lifespan Gap will be nearly nonexistent. And he hasn't done anything special other than stay active and live well. Science bears this out. A 2024 study of nearly 3,700 people found that movement, not just exercise but staying active each day, was the biggest predictor of longevity.[5] You move, you live.

So we're not "biohacking" anything here. We're not spending big money on untested medical theories and procedures.

I'm about getting out there and moving and having fun.

I'm about preserving and improving fitness, strength, mobility, balance, and flexibility.

I'm about preventing disease and increasing vitality through the science-tested power of physical activity.

I'm about improving mental health through movement.

I'm about preventing and working around injury.

Sweat is simple and well earned. And so are exercise's benefits.

Don't make it any more complicated than that.

Here's What Being in Love with Movement Looks Like

Flash back with me to an ordinary Saturday morning in New York City in January 2021. Prime time pandemic. It's sunny out, but about twenty-five degrees. Through my IronStrength community ties, I set up a one-hour, socially distanced outdoor workout in Central Park. High-intensity total-body strength training, all fitness levels welcome. I didn't care if two people showed up. I wanted to be out in the air in an open space.

More than *one hundred people* showed up. It was January, it was freezing, but a massive group came out anyway. What motivated them? At that hour on a winter morning my main competition for their attention was a warm bed and blanket—and my cold-weather workout won. How? I think it was being cooped up, for one. That made movement feel necessary for them, attractive, enticing, a *release* to get outside and move even in the cold. But more important, I think it was the sense of community and shared experience. We worked out in the freezing cold, got the air in our lungs, and stayed safely distanced the whole time. *We did that together.*

Those are the motivational phenomena that fascinate me. Why them? Why then? What can I do to replicate this in larger settings across distance and with lots more people?

How do I convince you to feel like that if you don't get moving you might just burst?

That's why we're here right now. In the end, I have to be better than a doctor to my patients—including my new "reader patients" like you who picked up this book. I eventually boiled down what I learned into a very simple rule:

Keep the patient pointed in the right direction.

If I do that, I'm better than just a healer. And my patients—and everyone they touch—are better for it. The world becomes a better place.

That's what I'm going to do here: give you the tools you need to realize your own love for movement once again.

So What Will This Book Accomplish?

I'm going to simplify movement for you. In fact, I'll make it so easy you'll feel silly for not giving it a try.

We'll focus on three things.

First, I'll help you understand the roots of healthy and unhealthy motivation, how they affect what you do each day, and how to change your choices for the better. Consistent, healthy motivation comes from an intertwining of knowledge, belief, and emotion.

Knowledge: *I should do this.*

Emotion: *I want to do this.*

Belief: *I can do this.*

While they combine in different amounts for each person, it's virtually impossible to make meaningful, lasting motivational change without all three.

Second, I'll help you determine your weak spots and where and how you can improve them. I've created a self-test that you can use again and again to track your motivational progress.

Third, I'll give you a four-week (and more if you choose) movement plan that will help you push through periods of difficulty with motivation and help you fall in love with movement again. This includes about eighty specific muscle-building exercises, infinite workout possibilities (I'll show you how to build your own!), and get-in-gear boosts along the way.

We've only scratched the surface here. We're going to dig a lot deeper and find out why your brain pushes you to do so many unhealthy things.

Oh, and congratulations. By opening this book, you've just done the mental equivalent of tying your sneakers and walking out the door for a twenty-five-degree morning workout in Central Park with one hundred of your closest workout buddies. You're going to learn how to push yourself when no one is looking. And you're going to fall in love all over again. Let's get started!

Jordan D. Metzl, MD
SPORTS MEDICINE
HOSPITAL FOR SPECIAL SURGERY
NEW YORK, NEW YORK

PART ONE

Rediscovering Movement

CHAPTER 1

What Is Movement?

If you asked me what movement means to me, to describe it so even a child could understand, I would start by saying this: Movement means to me exactly the same things it means to you.

There is no difference between me, a sports medicine physician who competes in triathlons and leads fitness classes, and you. Movement is the same for every human being.

This chapter, part science, part emotion, part experience, is the best explanation of movement I know.

Movement Is Life

It would be easy for me to say something glib like "If you ain't movin', you ain't livin'," but there's truth in that cheesy statement, both literally and metaphorically.

How does a medical professional determine a human being is alive? Movement. Chest up and down from respiration. Vibrations in the chest and wrist and throat from a pumping heart and flowing blood. Pupillary response when light hits the eyes. In a hospital setting, numbers on monitors rise and fall, ECGs illustrate cardiac activity (activity being movement), EEGs measure brain activity, and those old-school blood pressure cuffs have a hand pump and a needle jumping all around a circular gauge.

What do doctors say in certain situations when a patient is unconscious? *Squeeze my hand* or *wiggle your toes*. And what's one of the first things those wonderful hospital pros will have you do as soon as possible after a surgery or trauma or enough healing has happened?

Get up and move. Stand. Go to the toilet on your own. Walk down the hall and back. Bathe.

In my own practice, I often ask patients to move their limbs in a variety of ways, depending on their injury, so I can assess how severe the problem may be.

Movement is foundational to everything human beings do, to who and what we are.

Movement is the ordinary—taking laundry upstairs, chasing a toddler, pushing a mower—intertwining with the extraordinary—giving birth, crossing a finish line, a heart beating for more than ninety years straight.

It's foundational: the very bedrock of our lives, on the same level as eating, sleeping, and breathing. And it's perhaps even *more* foundational than those three things, since moving with purpose each day makes all your eating, sleeping, and breathing more efficient and healthier.

When you abandon movement, your life's foundation deteriorates. It is as inevitable as water seeping into cracks in concrete.

Think back to the three-year-old. The time when movement meant joy.

When we stop moving, the joy dies. We die.

Movement Is Medicine

I'm a doctor who regularly prescribes physical activity to my patients. Movement is by far the best medicine I know—so much so that I joined forces with colleagues from the Hospital for Special Surgery to create one of the first seminars to teach medical students, physicians of the future, how to prescribe exercise for their patients. Our seminar, "Prescribing the Medicine of Movement," is now required curriculum for second-year medical students at Cornell Medical School.

Why not say "Movement is health"? Because not everyone is healthy, but they can still move. People with injuries, limitations, and disabilities can move in different ways to make themselves stronger. Movement itself is not health—it is a sign of health and can be the path to better health. That's what I prescribe, that's what I aid and abet, that's what I see every day.

This medicine is also free, requires no trip to the pharmacy and no insurance company sign-off, has no negative side effects (sore muscles don't count, sorry), and can be taken as often as you like (infinite refills!). Oh, and if you take this medicine regularly, you eventually may be able to decrease or stop taking other medications for health issues that improve. That's right: More of this medicine can sometimes lead to less of other medicines.

How many health problems can movement help address? The actual number may not be known, but here's a sampling: heart disease, dementia/Alzheimer's, certain cancers, osteoarthritis, depression (exercise has long been known as "nature's antidepressant"), type 2 diabetes, prediabetes/metabolic syndrome, fatty liver, hypertension, high cholesterol, autoimmune disorders, osteopenia/osteoporosis, ADHD, sleep apnea, anxiety, asthma, menopause symptoms, low back pain, erectile dysfunction, stress, and more.[1] We are now learning that these changes in body systems described above correlate to cellular changes: maintaining telomeric length, improving mitochondrial volume and function, even reducing genomic instability. These types of cellular changes provide an even-greater appreciation of the major health benefits from moving every day. The changes that we can see, and the changes happening inside our cells, are profound.

Let's simplify this further. The biggest health threat we face isn't cancer or heart disease. It's low fitness. A sedentary life—the life more and more of us are living—promotes all diseases. A growing pile of research shows that low fitness causes more premature deaths than smoking, obesity, and high blood pressure. And very little exercise is required to achieve benefits. In one study of 334,000 Europeans, the people who enjoyed the greatest benefits of exercise—a 16 to 30 percent drop in mortality risk—were the ones who went from inactive to moderately inactive.[2] This doesn't mean you're running a marathon; it means you're getting out and doing something active for about half an hour a day.

EXERCISE IS MEDICINE FOR
HIGH BLOOD PRESSURE

A 2023 meta-analysis of 270 studies covering sixteen thousand people in the *British Journal of Sports Medicine* found that physical activity had a significant improvement on blood pressure.[3]

- People with normal blood pressure saw benefits, but those with hypertension saw the largest improvement in blood pressure.
- All forms of exercise tested were effective: aerobic, strength training, combined aerobic/strength training, high-intensity interval training (HIIT), and isometric training (grip strength, leg extensions, wall squats).
- Isometric exercises were most effective. Why? Researchers suggest that movements like wall squats, where you hold in the seated position for an extended period, involve longer muscle contraction, which can reduce blood flow in the muscles. When the muscles relax, blood rushes back in causing a process called "reactive hyperemia," which produces nitric oxide in the body and relaxes blood vessels. Over time, this can improve blood pressure.
- One last pretty important detail: Exercise has been shown to be comparable to medication in reducing blood pressure.

Why is inactivity so destructive? Many reasons, all bad. The pandemic ripped away the curtains on a number of societal problems we haven't addressed, and one of the biggest is our low fitness and poor physical condition in general. The most damaging comorbidities of COVID-19 are obesity and its associated health problems, plus a lethal attraction to our lungs. People with deconditioned lungs and unmanaged weight-related health issues had more severe infections and higher death rates. People who were in better physical condition fared better.

But COVID was new. The problems the virus capitalized on have been with us for decades. So let's focus on one of the worst. Aside from your muscles and joints deteriorating from lack of use, lack of activity means you unavoidably gain weight. That weight gain, particularly in your midsection, is dangerous.

I mentioned "inflammaging" before. Do you know what chronic low-grade inflammation is and does? Inflammation itself is an immune system response. Red swelling around a sprained ankle is an example of acute, short-term inflammation. So are your runny nose and irritated eyes during a head cold. Your body's immune system is working to heal these short-term maladies. With COVID, inflammation sometimes goes off the charts, and that alone can be life-threatening. Our immune systems are designed to remember certain illnesses we've had—but *no one* had had COVID-19. Crazy immune response, crazy inflammation levels. And the virus and inflammation can linger in the brain, lungs, spinal fluid, and more to cause long COVID for months or years. But to return to my initial point: That garden-variety inflammation resolves in days when the sprained ankle improves or when the cold runs its course.

When you have low-grade chronic inflammation, the immune response doesn't stop. Always running a little hot, always on—and you usually never know. All that chronic inflammation causes damage. The condition is linked to most serious diseases, particularly the deadliest: heart disease, cancer, dementia/Alzheimer's, type 2 diabetes, autoimmune disorders, and many more. (Seeing a pattern here vis-à-vis exercise and the diseases it can help prevent?)

What elevates chronic inflammation? The joys of a sedentary life: poor diet, excess weight, unmanaged stress, lousy sleep, and smoking/drinking. Getting older too, and what happens as we age? For most people, weight gain and lower activity levels.

Know what else causes inflammation? Inflammation. Chronic immune response can promote weight gain. And fat, especially visceral belly fat that lives in and around organs like your liver, is a highly inflammatory tissue in itself. It's metabolically active—and not in a nice way. Every day, your belly fat releases inflammatory compounds into your body (compounds with Bond-villain names like *interleukin-6* and *tumor necrosis factor-alpha*), which are linked to insulin resistance and make inflammation worse. So, in a twisted physiological joke, inflammation makes belly fat that tries to make more belly fat by triggering more inflammation.[4]

What can help lower inflammation levels? Movement. Want to lower your inflammation levels *immediately*? Take a brisk walk. One 2017 study found lower inflammatory blood markers in participants after just twenty minutes on a treadmill.[5] Want to lower your inflammation levels long term? Keep walking.

Exercise and inflammation work like this: You do a workout, your short-term inflammation levels rise, then resolve, and the long-term result is lower overall inflammation levels.[6] This is true of low- and high-intensity activity over short periods with normal recovery (though more extreme long-form exercise with improper recovery can hurt immune function—the vast majority of people do not have to worry about this).

Building and maintaining muscle—extending your musclespan— also has anti-inflammatory and endocrine-like benefits. Muscle secretes myokines that act as messengers between many organs and help facilitate positive functions.[7] This is why natural muscle and strength loss from aging, sarcopenia and dynapenia, can be so damaging as you get older.

The more you move long term, the more muscle you maintain, the lower your inflammation levels, the healthier you become, and the lower your overall risk for serious disease.

There are dozens of ways movement is medicine. That's one.

If you're unhealthy, use movement to get healthier.
If you're healthy, use movement to stay that way.

I can continue to throw research at you, and will, but in the end, this is an emotional issue. Much has been written about the medical advantages movement brings you (I wrote an entire book on it, *The Exercise Cure;* the science is deep and definitive), but none of it matters if you don't take the information to heart. We'll talk a lot more in the coming chapters about how information intertwines with your emotions, but if you can't accept one of the most basic and proven aspects of medicine—movement is good for you—you doom yourself to health problems you may otherwise never have if you remain active.

Movement Is Life Altering

There are two ways to take the term *life altering.*

You can go with the day-to-day meaning: I started exercising regularly and my life changed for the better. All manner of changes, all types of lives. I ran that marathon or climbed that mountain or stopped falling asleep at my desk at 3 P.M. I met someone amazing, my back stopped hurting, I no longer need my CPAP. Think of all the real-people examples in your own life.

Movement is metamorphic. If you take up regular physical activity and stay with it, I guarantee your life will change for the better.

The second meaning of *life altering* is the same, but also different. Movement will change you, of course, but not like you normally think.

What are the building blocks of life? Our cells. And regular physical activity can alter our cellular function in positive ways. Yes, exercise can transform you all the way down to your cells.

Example: The energy factories within your cells are called the mitochondria. They produce energy your cells need to function. A study in *Frontiers of Physiology* examined proteins that help fuel mitochondria in muscle cells—more than four thousand proteins were identified.[8] That's not the cool part. People who exercised regularly produced more of these proteins to fuel cellular function in muscle. The long answer: Bad things like DNA damage and senescence (cell death) were lower in the muscle cells of active people, essentially slowing the muscular aging process. And this was true at most any age (participants ranged in age from twenty to eighty-seven). Also, the physical activity involved was basic, "not intense competitive exercise," so anyone can do it. The short answer: Being active can slow aging on a cellular level.

There's more. A 2023 study in *Aging Cell* examined genome data in two groups of sedentary people (ages forty to sixty-five).[9] One group did nothing. But the participants who did three twenty-three-minute sessions of high-intensity interval training (HIIT) each week for four weeks showed a transcriptomatic (looking at RNA molecules in cells) age reduction of 3.6 years, with a 3.3-year increase in the inactive group. HIIT exercisers' age-related gene expression changed for the better.

Researchers have also examined genetic aspects of physical activity (specifically, genes called alleles that occur on our chromosomes) and found that genes associated with movement/exercise are older than we are[10]—as in, Neanderthals had the same physical activity genes we do today. Movement is ingrained in us on a cellular level. We're made that way. We're *supposed* to move.

Exercise science has made big strides toward finding how physical activity whips our cells into shape. Putting this in very general terms, exercise stresses the body, and then the body recovers—so physical activity effectively trains the body to better handle stressors. This helps improve healthspan and extend lifespan. We touched on inflammation already, and more research is under way. For example, MoTrPAC (Molecular Transducers of Physical Activity Consortium), a large ten-year research project doing deep dives into how physical activity "improves health and prevents disease," continues to add more data to a growing pile. Some of their 2024 studies found that endurance exercise triggered positive effects throughout the body across immune, metabolic, stress response, and mitochondrial pathways (ongoing research in rats and humans, with more human data to come).[11] As the researchers write, it comes down to this: "We hypothesize that by subjecting the body to disease-like stresses, regular exercise elicits adaptation to the symptoms of those diseases, reducing the risk of their manifestation from the disease itself."

Then there's this: Our chromosomes exist as long strings with caps on their tips called telomeres (I've heard the comparison that telomeres are like the plastic tips of your shoelaces). As your cells die over time, your telomeres gradually become shorter. Just a natural result of the aging we all experience, right? Yes, but it's not completely out of our control. Some research suggests that being physically active slows down the shortening of your telomeres. In effect, exercise may slow the aging process on a cellular level. A *Preventive*

Medicine study of 5,800 adults doing sixty-two physical activities compared sedentary people and "high-activity" people and found that the active folks had a nine-year aging advantage over the folks who did nothing.[12] But amounts count too. The aging difference between "moderate" activity and "high" activity was 7.1 years.

This is the essence of what I mean when I talk about longevity. A lot of new science has emerged looking at our "biological age" versus our chronological age (how many birthdays we've had). Biological age is how old you are on a cellular level, and not everyone is the same. If you want to know your biological age, that's currently hard to pin down because it's difficult to get accurate readings on, say, your telomere length, or to see how your body handles a process called DNA methylation, or to access a really good epigenetic clock (spoiler alert: No one can, though consumers will in the future). But over and over again, research shows that regular exercisers have a biological aging advantage over those who are sedentary, especially when you add in other lifestyle factors like healthy eating and quality sleep, and when you see elsewhere in this book about how exercise is good for XYZ medical condition or healthspan or musclespan, it all ties together: longevity. That's what it's all about.

You don't have to spend huge amounts of money on anything fancy, experimental, or quasi-scientific to improve your biological age. You want a fountain of youth? Rise up from the sofa. Tie your sneakers and walk out the door.

Movement Is Cumulative

By now you've heard all the benchmarks for physical activity. "Get your ten thousand steps!" Hey, why not? That's about five miles of walking. Then you have the U.S. government recommendations of 150 minutes of moderate-intensity physical activity per week.[13] That shakes out to about 22 minutes of brisk walking a day. But wait— that's the minimum. The guidelines actually say 150 to 300 minutes per week.

Wow, people say, *150 minutes. Sounds like a lot. And 300 minutes? That's five hours! Heck with that.*

Oh, there are variations on the weekly recs. Intensity matters. If you ramp up the effort—like with running or a more intense sport—the recs drop to 75 to 150 minutes per week. So, you go out for a 30-minute run three or four times a week and you're there.

There's more: The guidelines recommend adding two sessions of strength training per week to boot.

There's still more: The guidelines say if you do *more* than all that, your health benefits increase—which reinforces what I've been telling you so far.

All of this creates a big problem—one that has an attractive solution.

The problem: Folks see those hefty 150 and 300 numbers and balk. Those numbers just feel like a lot, even if you break them down to daily amounts. Exercising every single day can feel like a lot for some people too.

The solution: Break it all up even further. One thing no one talks much about with these guidelines is that movement is cumulative. Everything you do each day adds up. Take a five-minute walk around the block at 10 A.M., another twelve-minute stroll at lunch, and another ten-minute jaunt after dinner. Suddenly you're pushing thirty minutes for the day.

And what about what researchers call "vigorous intermittent lifestyle physical activity" (VILPA)? Think of household chores done at a good pace. A UK study in *Nature Medicine* of more than twenty-five thousand "nonexercisers" with a mean age of sixty-two found that those who had at least three one- to two-minute bursts of VILPA every day had up to a 30 percent reduction in cancer mortality risk and a 34 percent reduction in cardiovascular disease mortality risk.[14] Oh, and studying nearly sixty-five thousand exercisers found similar results.

Another 2022 study in the *European Heart Journal* followed nearly seventy-two thousand people over a median of six years and found that even short bursts of "vigorous physical activity" reduced risk of heart disease death.[15] The minimal dose was about fifteen minutes per week, or about two minutes per day. And the more people did, the lower their risk.

More evidence: In 2020, University of Texas researchers had study participants interrupt a normally sedentary eight-hour period with four-second bursts of high-intensity stationary cycling five times an hour over a workday.[16] That's two minutes, forty seconds of exercise total. That small amount of intermittent activity over a workday brought people fat oxidation benefits lasting into the following day.

These are sometimes called exercise "snacks."

Why do you think all those smartphone and smartwatch manufacturers include all those activity tracking apps? So you can see the step count, the stairs you climb, the number of times you stand, all the little things you do that *accumulate* into a daily total.

Small doses add up, and all movement matters.

Movement Is for All—and Especially for You

After meeting and treating and working with thousands of people, I can say this: Everyone is different, everyone sees different things, everyone wants different things, everyone is who they are.

Some people have easier lives than others.

Some people have fewer obstacles than others.

Not everyone is as sensitive to other people's needs as they could be.

Not everyone treats everyone the same.

People make assumptions about other people.

But everyone moves.

Movement is neutral. Movement doesn't judge. Movement doesn't assume. Movement meets you right where you are and asks, "Where would you like to go?"

Everyone has some kind of healthy movement they can do, want to do, or have the potential to do.

Everyone can improve. Any physical condition, any age, anytime, anyplace.

No matter what other people say, do, or think—you can move.

Movement allows you to leave all the negative people behind.

Movement Is a Statement

You know the old saying: Actions speak louder than words. So, what are you saying with movement? Because you make a statement when you commit to moving with purpose every day. Why? Well, the way I see it, we have a low-fitness epidemic in our culture. People who choose regular physical activity as a part of their lives really are making a decision that pushes back on all the things that conspire to keep us inactive. That's bold. So I truly believe a person makes a statement—conscious or unconscious, nonverbal or verbal—when they choose movement. Here's mine:

"I love how daily physical activity makes me feel. Movement has always helped me. Throughout my life, no matter what challenge I faced in my career or elsewhere, I always performed better at my job, at my relationships, at everything, when I was physically active. I am committed to my own fitness and healthspan, and I am committed to those of my patients, loved ones, and all the people I have never met who might benefit from what I know. That's why I'm here. That's why I do it."

I don't say this out loud, of course, but every day I represent this statement.

I've had a long time to think about why I stay moving. Your statement doesn't have to be nearly as detailed, nor do you even have to verbalize it or write it down. It can be just a thought: *I'm done with lying around. I'm ready to do more.* But anytime you're on the move, you'll know it.

Maybe your statement sounds something like these:

I'm adding life to my years and years to my life. My healthspan is just as important to me, if not more, than my lifespan.

I'm making the world a better place with my health. It keeps me active and engaged with everyone I know and love, and we all benefit from our varying communities.

Movement is not my favorite thing, and that's okay. But I'm doing it anyway because I'm motivated to feel healthier and live longer.

Everything about my day is better when I move. I want to feel better at work, perform better, and be mentally sharper.

I move because no one can do it for me. I move because I never regret it afterward.

I want to know what I am capable of.

I'm strong. But I could be stronger.

We could make a granite wall as tall and long as a New York City block and still not have enough room to carve all the possible statements into that stone.

Movement Is Magic

I won't get all metaphysical on you. But movement is spiritual; it is happiness, it is positivity, it lifts you up.

Movement is transformative. It changes your body for the better—strength, flexibility, balance, endurance, overall physical ability. Your mind then transforms along with it—elevated mood, better focus, positive feelings of direction and accomplishment. And those changes usually happen quickly and continue to build over time.

Movement is improvement. Physical activity can preserve and prevent, but for most people, it is the road to better.

Movement is challenge. Can you push harder? Can you stick with it even when everything in your brain says, "Skip it"?

Movement is revealing. You say you want to exercise more, get in shape, run a race, look better naked—so why haven't you? Movement, and the refusal of movement, tells the real story.

Movement is foolproof. It is, and will always be, the one thing we can use and trust to elevate ourselves: our health, our mood, our abilities, our perspective, our optimism, our appetite for living. Movement can be as simple or complex as we want. It can be as easy or intense as we want. We control how, when, where, and why we move. It's not just the key to your optimum life, it's the keychain. It's not just a tool for elevation, it's the toolshed.

It's so simple.

Movement is everything.

CHAPTER 2

Push Yourself

How many times in your life has someone said to you, "Push yourself!" The person saying it can be well-intentioned, or impatient, or frustrated. And so can you be, the person who has to hear it. Because the underlying message is clear: You're not good enough, doing enough, fast enough.

"Push yourself" is many things: a cliché, a criticism, and, when you hear it often enough, meaningless.

Let's make the word *push* a positive from here on out. When you read it in this book, I want you to feel warm intention in your belly. Anticipation for better. Ammunition for achievement. Pushing yourself has to become the more attractive option because, let's be honest here, all this time you haven't been pushing yourself has taken a toll.

"Push yourself" from now on means progress. Activation. Positivity. A step from unhealthy toward healthy, from sadness to joy.

This isn't a pep talk. This is important and the first actual bit of work you have to do for this book: internalizing that the word *push* is positive. This all has to do with emotion, which is a key ingredient in healthy motivation. It also has to do with perception, how you feel about something you hear or see. Changing how you perceive things, you'll soon see, is how you change everything.

maybe we don't talk about how we don't do the actual movement, but boy, do we love watching others do the actual movement. We admire from a distance those who dance well, or family and friends who run races or do front knocks off the diving board, or who can roll that basketball from fingertip to fingertip while weaving between overaggressive cousins and neighbors. "My grandfather still does hill sprints. Hill sprints!" We cheer for all our sports every day. We watch the pros and elite college athletes on TV and in stadiums. We tune into the Olympics to watch the most unique sports put the true beauty of human movement on display (if figure skating is physical poetry, then gymnastics is savage poetry, but poetry all the same). Locally, high school sports still draw more crowds and funding than the debate club. And parents still get into fistfights with other parents and volunteer refs during youth sports matches—all because of how kids move.

(The Olympics, in particular, have been studied to see how the Games positively or negatively affect physical activity rates in host cities and other communities. There's no evidence that watching the Olympics causes any increase in physical activity across the population, and hosting the Games doesn't inspire a city's population to become more active even though they're immersed in that culture for a time. So, yeah, they're inspiring to watch, but that inspiration seems to be confined to the couch.)[1]

We love movement. But many of us hate to do it ourselves. Why?

Tough question, hard answer. The easy answer: Blame your brain. But that may not be the simplest answer (easy and simple, I'm sure you've heard, are not the same). The fact is, there are a *lot* of reasons. The Western lifestyle pushes us toward unhealthy things, including an increasing reliance on technology that makes movement less necessary to work, to socialize, to exist. This has created tendencies, perceptions, and biases in us that sabotage our best intentions and overpower what we know to be the smarter, healthier action.

Walk with Me

Let's take a quick tour of what you're dealing with.

The world is, to put it mildly, messed up. The pandemic, to me, wasn't just a health crisis. It was a powerful magnifying glass that showed us just how unhealthy and unprepared we are for any widespread health threat. And like a magnifying glass on an anthill, it burned us.

The pandemic changed a few things for me, just as it probably has for you.

I've been thinking about motivation for years, in everything that I do. With COVID-19, the concept of keeping my patients and community healthy and on track—when the entire world was off the rails—brought this issue into a clearer light for me.

By every known metric, our society grew more sedentary, gained more weight, and became less healthy during the pandemic. Stress levels rose and mental health declined. Loved ones died. For a long time, we were stuck in our homes. For months we depended on our computers for work, news, and socialization. We had no physical outlet. Gyms shut down. For a while, even outdoor parks were closed. You will never see an actual stat on this, but imagine the collective number of hangovers between March 2020 and today. COVID-19 is still with us. Long COVID is real and can be debilitating. It's been a demoralizing and depressing time that *continues* to take a toll on all of us.

I think there were a lot of poorly motivated people before the pandemic. I think the trauma of the pandemic produced even more.

One notable and sobering piece of research: A September 2022 study in *PLOS One* found that the pandemic may have changed aspects of our personalities—and not in a good way.[2] More than seven thousand people participated, answering questions in February 2020 and then again in 2021 and 2022. Results: negative impacts on five personality areas—neuroticism, extroversion, openness, agreeableness, and conscientiousness. Young adults in the study were especially susceptible to "disrupted maturity." Now understand that, as the study authors say, these five areas are considered by researchers to be "relatively impervious to environmental demands in adulthood"—which means they change very little over time. The two-year shift in this study represented what would normally be *a decade* of change.

But who are we kidding? The pandemic was an extreme event, for sure, but from a public health standpoint, we were already on a bad road. A 2019 study in *The New England Journal of Medicine*—published before the pandemic—examined health and weight data going back to 1993, and researchers predict that one out of two Americans will have obesity by 2030.[3] Not just excess weight—obesity. They also predict that 25 percent of adults will have *severe* obesity, prevalence will be higher than 50 percent in twenty-nine U.S. states, and no states will have obesity rates below 35 percent.

Right now, more than one in ten Americans has type 2 diabetes (thirty-eight million people), according to the American Diabetes Association.[4] Another ninety-six million have prediabetes through a condition known as metabolic syndrome. Together that's more than half of all American adults suffering from a deadly health condition brought on primarily by lifestyle—poor diet and being sedentary. Diabetes is our most expensive disease.

Nine in ten

Estimated number of Americans who can be considered "metabolically unhealthy" (87.8 percent)

Metabolic health = optimal levels of waist circumference, fasting glucose, blood pressure, triglycerides, high-density lipoprotein (HDL) cholesterol, and not taking any related medication.[5]

And the lack of physical fitness overall is, well, pick your adjective. Stunning. Disturbing. In a 2022 study that looked at how older adults received care, researchers uncovered stats from the National Center for Health Statistics' National Health Interview Survey showing that nearly one in ten people age forty-five to sixty-four in the United States were frail and another 22 percent pre-frail (defined by weakness and low fitness, something more commonly seen in very old adults).[6] Meanwhile, 51 percent of people age sixty-five or older qualified as frail or pre-frail. It's disturbing to imagine a forty- or fifty-something person as *frail,* but here we are.

This data shows a serious falling out of love with physical activity on a nationwide scale.

(Cue an overzealous coach screaming, "Why can't you just push yourselves!")

"Push" is positive now, remember?

Let's rise out of the negative into the positive.

If you can absorb what's coming in this book and learn to push yourself—positively, ambitiously, enthusiastically—a lot of what you just read won't be an issue for you any longer.

Time for Some Good Stuff

So, all those bad stats, how did that happen? How did we get to that place? And how can we possibly be positive about it? Well, we need to bring the big, broad statistics down to an individual level and begin highlighting what turns motivation negative—and by "individual," I mean *you*.

It's rarely one cause. It's usually a cocktail of causes.

What are they? Where do they come from? What makes them so powerful?

The next section of the book will dive deep into these causes and show you how they work. I guarantee you'll see yourself in there as we go, maybe one or two primary issues, maybe a whole bunch.

You need to have a solid understanding of these causes and then you can target them. By the time you reach the four-week plan and other take-control things later in the book, you will have come to understand what I call "the Big List." Each item on the list represents a major factor in healthy/unhealthy motivation, and we'll discuss them all in detail. My goal is to help you recognize how each factor on this list affects your motivation and, by mastering them, learn how to push yourself.

Here's the Big List:

1. Biases
2. Perception
3. Incentives
4. Knowledge
5. Curiosity
6. Self-esteem
7. Self-efficacy
8. Control

9. Community

10. (It's a secret!)

Don't worry, you don't have to memorize them; you'll be seeing them again. But have a look, and you start to see a path come into focus. As we move through each one, you'll find yourself saying, "Oh yeah, that's me" on a variety of levels. And those realizations will all come to bear when it's time for you to truly make positive change.

The 60 Percent Solution

Let's talk about healthspan again. My patient Alice is the gold standard of long healthspan. Kettlebells in your eighties—I dare you to do better.

Where does a longer healthspan come from? What I call the "60 percent." It goes like this:

Science tells us our genes determine roughly 25 percent of the variation in the human lifespan.[7] That basically means your parents aren't fully responsible for your incoming heart attack (sorry, can't blame them for everything).

Science also tells us that medical care can account for only 10 to 20 percent of the "modifiable contributors" to healthy outcomes in a given population.[8] That means your doctor can help you try to prevent that heart attack, and treat you when it happens, but the endgame can't be predicted.

That leaves us with approximately 60 percent (give or take) of other things determining your healthspan. Public health researchers call these other things "social determinants of health."[9] So it's all the other stuff outside of genetics and medical care that makes you who you are and your health what it is.

Some of that is your environment—where you live, air/water quality, availability of healthy resources, public safety. That's not always in your control. The rest of that is your lifestyle, for lack of a better word, and it's all the stuff you can push yourself to control: what you eat, how often you move, how much you sleep, how you manage stress, how much booze you drink, what recreational drugs you enjoy, how many positive social interactions you have, how much you educate yourself (not just from formal schooling), and how many packs a day you smoke.

That's where we're working in this book: the things in the 60 percent you control.

Lifespan, Healthspan, and Musclespan

As we learn more about the concepts of lifespan and healthspan, we are increasingly recognizing the importance of *musclespan:* how long you're able to maintain your skeletal muscle mass across your lifespan. *Strengthspan* is another element, your strength across time. It's all critical to long-term health.

We think of muscle as the organ that moves our skeleton and protects our joints and organs (and makes us look great naked). From a sports medicine perspective, this is largely how we've thought for decades. However, we've touched on some of this already: Muscle can also be thought of as a large and powerful endocrine gland. Your muscles hold the largest store of glucose in the body, and maintaining muscle, particularly skeletal muscle, across the lifespan is an essential marker of not only how you move but how metabolically capable you are. As such, the three components of longevity include lifespan, healthspan, and musclespan (with a nod to strengthspan too). In the second half of this book, we'll talk about ways to maximize your musclespan throughout your life, particularly as you age and as metabolic function declines. Excess glucose in the blood is a poison, and our body spends tremendous amounts of energy removing it, converting it, and storing it. The more muscle we have, the better we're able to store it; it's like having extra gigabytes on your computer. So along with strength and fitness, that's why a long, well-maintained musclespan is so important.

Unfortunately, muscle doesn't build itself.

You want to feel great today? Next week? Next decade?

Push yourself.

And Let's Be Specific About What "Push Yourself" Means

I also want you to understand that in this book, "Push yourself" means mentally *and* physically. They go hand in hand because most people have to push themselves up here (taps head) before they get moving. Push your mind, push your body. And what we're really pushing for is better mental and physical health intertwined to make you feel and behave healthier.

I was lucky; I lived this growing up. My dad was a pediatrician, my mom a psychologist, so that dual approach—physical and mental—was in the water at home, and I grew up thinking about health in both ways. Therefore, when we start thinking about a topic like fitness motivation and pushing, understand that we're training mind and body here. By pushing the mind, you're better able to push the body, and by pushing the body, you are training your mind for healthier future motivation.

Also important: This is about learning to push your mind and body to a place where both are a little bit uncomfortable. Think of each positive step as the next step up a ladder. I think about this a lot from my own speed training. I'll do a series of six half-mile sprints, and I hate it while I'm doing it and feel like I'm going to puke. But I also know that I *need* this discomfort and need to push through it, because when I'm done, I get all the benefits: I feel physically great head to toe and mentally great for making the effort. When I get back to my distance training, I run stronger and faster.

Push mind, push body, push yourself. That's how this works.

Loves Movement, Hates to Move

Here's an interesting phenomenon: Our society appears to simultaneously be obsessed with fitness while having never been more sedentary and unhealthy.

Evidence: Millions of us who are sedentary still worship movement every single day. Maybe we don't do the actual movement,

CHAPTER 3

Motivation Is a Big Word

So let's answer a fundamental question. *The* fundamental question. *Why is it so hard for so many of us to keep moving?*

That joy of moving just for the fun of it has evaporated. The love affair is over. What happened?

There are several answers—and they all connect to one thing: motivation.

To that point, the first thing you see when you walk into my office is a sign on the wall:

> *The medicine of movement*
> *is one of the most powerful forms of*
> *preventive health.*
> *It works for everyone who takes it,*
> *young and old alike.*

Age, gender, race, sexual orientation, political inclination, religion, Yankees or Red Sox, Elvis or Beatles, whichever way you replace a roll of toilet paper *do not matter.* Whether you're trying to walk with your grandkids or make the school baseball team, I want you thinking about that quote. In fact, that quote is right there when patients come into my office. I'm always trying to keep my patients pointed in the right direction, and the quote is one more piece of motivation, one more push. In my lectures I always say, "The Holy Grail of exercise is compliance": doing that work, day in, day out, over months and years. And the Holy Grail of compliance is *motivation*.

Motivation is a loaded word.

Yes, it drives us to do things. But you hear people all the time say, "I just don't have the motivation today." "Totally unmotivated, LOL." "Yeah, it ain't happening today." A hundred versions of the same declaration: I don't feel interested in doing the best things for myself today.

But we get something wrong about motivation that interferes with our understanding of it. We associate the word only with positive actions—as in, you have to be motivated to go for a run, or make a salad, or drive to the gym. That's where all those "I'm so unmotivated" people come from.

Here's a thought: You are never, not for one second, ever without motivation. You're human—you are *perpetually* motivated. The problems start when motivation drives you to do unhealthy things.

"Lack of motivation"

The number one barrier to physical activity reported by people with obesity, according to a 2021 review of twenty-seven studies in *PLOS One*.[1]

The Ins(ides) and Outs(ides) of What Drives You

There are two kinds of motivation. Richard Ryan and Edward Deci, psychologists and professors, described it this way in a paper more than twenty years ago: People "can be urged into action by an abiding interest or by a bribe."[2]

That about sums up *intrinsic* and *extrinsic* motivation (some use the terms *autonomous* and *controlled*).

Intrinsic motivation comes from within. You desire to do something because you love it, you're curious, or you want to see a certain outcome.

Extrinsic motivation happens when some outside force drives you to do something: a reward, a responsibility, a law or contract, or some other form of enticement or coercion.

When you think of your three-year-old self running around and jumping and playing, you're the poster child for intrinsic motivation. You're moving all the time because you want to: Your inner drive pushes you all over the place at full speed. You love it. However, intrinsic motivation can also be the force driving you to skip workouts later in life, to hug the couch, to eat and drink things that give you pleasure now and pain later. Intrinsic motivation can be good or bad for you. Some people truly desire to live in a healthy way and use that positive motivation to their benefit without needing outside help. A majority of others have intrinsic motivation to do the opposite.

Extrinsic motivation works both ways too. Maybe some sort of outside influence pushes you to work in healthy ways—a coach, a mentor, a team, a loved one, or some nonperson like money, competition, a health threat, or even imitation because you want to look or perform like someone else. Case in point: A 2017 study from two MIT researchers followed a global network of 1.1 million runners over five years and found exercise to be socially contagious—the running habits of friends influenced other friends to run harder and longer.[3]

Outside factors can just as easily have you choosing unhealthy things—a similarly unhealthy partner, a drinking buddy or happy hour crew, or other forces like peer pressure, mental or physical health limitations, unregulated stress, or emotions tied to outside influences like anger, fear, and jealousy.

And how about this: Some people feel like exercise is all or nothing and if they can't do it the "right" way they won't bother. What is this mystical "right" way? I'm not sure. I've never heard of it. If you're moving and challenging your body, you're doing it right. But people perceive things in their own way, and not always the healthy way.

See how this works? *Motivation all the time.* It just depends on what kind of motivation is pushing you, and where to.

Truths:

- One can be motivated—to train for months to run a marathon or triathlon.
- One can be motivated—to take online courses at night to earn a master's degree.
- One can be motivated—to lie on the couch.
- One can be motivated—to eat four brown sugar cinnamon toaster pastries at 10 P.M. on a Tuesday.

You get the point. Motivation is constant. Your body and mind push you to do things. The *nature* of those things is what matters, and the nature of those things can change from hour to hour, even minute to minute. The flow of these motivations never stops. In that respect, motivation resembles a river. Always flowing, pushing in one direction, moving us forward to act. And that, my friends, is why it can be so difficult to maintain motivations in certain directions. Ever try to alter the course of a river?

Well, that's exactly what people who change their lives for the better do—despite a powerful motivational flow telling them to go in an unhealthy direction.

Let's take a look at your unique case.

What Throws You Off-Balance?

Motivation is not a zero-sum, win-or-lose proposition. I believe we all live on a motivational spectrum that remains ever fluid. Some days are better than others. Heck, some mornings are better than some afternoons. The spectrum looks like this:

healthy motivation—inconsistent middle ground—unhealthy motivation
|—sweet spot—occasional wins, just as many losses—harmful lifestyle—|

The sweet spot is not "perfect" motivation and "absolute" consistency. That doesn't exist. It's general consistency with your decisions and activity (which a lot of people have on the unhealthy end, consistently doing things against their own best interests).

What throws you off-balance? The same issues that helped determine where you exist on the spectrum—and what you may be up against when your body and brain push you in an unhealthy direction. Some are intrinsic (inside) and some extrinsic (outside). The following are very common:

- Previous unhealthy activity that creates an urge for more unhealthy activity (you're hungover and crave lousy food; you slept badly because of stress and want to skip your routine; you did something you feel guilty about)
- Physical condition (low fitness; injury; disability; autoimmune diseases; chronic conditions)
- Bad memories of physical activity in some form, for any number of reasons. Research has shown that people who associate a positive memory motivating them to exercise were more likely to work out than the folks who had a negative memory association toward exercise.[4] This leads to a constant negative perception of all exercise: You don't like the way it makes you feel mentally and/or physically (a good reason to try to score some positive exercise experiences ASAP).
- You just don't like physical activity anymore because of the reasons I just mentioned, or others. Plus, it requires effort, time, and everything else you find unappealing right now.
- Life challenges (work/career; unforeseen accident/event; a pandemic; the news cycle)
- Family and friends (peer pressure; parenting/caregiving stress; lack of time for self)
- Mental health (perhaps the biggest issue because all of the above affect it, and vice versa; this includes diagnosable conditions and/or emotional state of mind)

Is the goal to reach the "sweet spot" on the spectrum? It can be. But overall improvement can be good enough.

That's why my goal for you as we make our way through this book is twofold:

- First, move you toward the left side of that motivational spectrum and get you comfortable with pushing yourself when necessary.
- Second, give you the physical tools and know-how to support that healthy motivation.

"Become comfortable" is the key phrase there. See, I can tell you what to do: "Push yourself! Fall back in love with movement!" You might do it, you might not. But if you read through to the final chapter—and each chapter will be a positive step in that direction—you'll have a much deeper understanding of your own motivational profile, as well as a much deeper appreciation of what movement is and what it means to you. In other words, you'll know how you tick—and how to push back against lousy motivations.

Another way to look at it: You want to shift your thinking so that your intrinsic motivations are healthy more often than not, and you seek out extrinsic factors that have a positive impact on your choices while avoiding the negative ones.

SOME WANT THE FUTURE OF EXERCISE TO BE— NO EXERCISE

Medical science continues on a path to potentially limiting—or even eliminating—the need to exercise.

University of Florida researchers—and others worldwide—are working on a class of drugs called "exercise mimetics," a pharmacological way to mimic exertion in the body. They administered a new drug called SLU-PP-332 to obese mice that triggered energy expenditure and fatty acid oxidation while improving insulin sensitivity. The drug also increased their physical endurance without them having to exercise.[5]

A 2022 study in *Cell Metabolism* by Australian researchers found that a certain gene activated in humans after skeletal muscle contraction—aka from movement—may offer clues to replicating the physiological effects of exercise.[6] They were able to increase the strength response in a frog's leg via an exercise mimetic.

Meanwhile a 2023 study in *Nature* showed how researchers were able to generate new muscle in mice suffering from a form of muscular dystrophy by injecting them with muscle stem cells.[7] The regenerative therapy potential for this is obvious, as well as the potential for using new muscle tissue to help manage, for example, diabetes. We know muscle tissue can help absorb glucose from the blood, which is why strength training is so helpful for people with insulin resistance.

Now, the point of all this research—and the millions of dollars funding it—is to help treat people with conditions like obesity and/or type 2 diabetes or muscular dystrophy or even frailty in old age. That makes sense and is vital. But you just know someone will eventually market an "exercise pill" to a willing public. Otherwise-healthy people will rush to use these breakthroughs so they never have to exercise at all, or to mitigate a lifetime of sedentary behavior.

I say be careful what you wish for. It's always amazing to have new therapies for sick people who need them. But perpetuating the idea that one day we'll have "exercise in a pill" or lab-grown muscles only contributes to the negative attitude a lot of people have toward physical activity.

We need to embrace movement, not find ways to avoid it.

Self-Test: Find Out Where You Are on the Motivational Spectrum

I know you're here because you acknowledge you have unhealthy motivation issues. But how bad is it for you? Let's find a simple way to quantify it.

This self-test is by no means scientific, nor is it diagnostic. It is designed for two things. First, each item touches on a subject in this book, so you'll have more and more awareness of the things that affect your fitness motivation. Second, it gives you a snapshot of where you are today. When you finish reading the book and try the four-week plan in a later chapter, take this test again for another snapshot.

The goal is not perfection. The goal is improvement.

All you need for the test is five minutes and some first-grade math.

And of course, *honesty.* Answer each item honestly, add up your score, and see where your point total puts you on the motivational spectrum.

Here you go:

In a given week, I avoid or skip physical activity . . .

Never	Almost never	Seldom	Half the time	Usually	Almost always	Always
0	1	2	3	4	5	6

If no outside forces push me, I will choose a less healthy activity (such as skipping a workout).

Never	Almost never	Seldom	Half the time	Usually	Almost always	Always
0	1	2	3	4	5	6

I perceive healthy activities and my ability to do them in a negative way, which affects my motivation to do them.

Never	Almost never	Seldom	Half the time	Usually	Almost always	Always
0	1	2	3	4	5	6

Even though I know what healthy choices to make, I make unhealthy choices.

Never	Almost never	Seldom	Half the time	Usually	Almost always	Always
0	1	2	3	4	5	6

I excuse or justify my unhealthy choices.

Never	Almost never	Seldom	Half the time	Usually	Almost always	Always
0	1	2	3	4	5	6

I believe I am capable of more in life but do not take action to improve.

Never	Almost never	Seldom	Half the time	Usually	Almost always	Always
0	1	2	3	4	5	6

I make unhealthy choices when I am alone.

Never	Almost never	Seldom	Half the time	Usually	Almost always	Always
0	1	2	3	4	5	6

I do not seek out people or groups that could help me make healthier choices.

Never	Almost never	Seldom	Half the time	Usually	Almost always	Always
0	1	2	3	4	5	6

I am envious of people I see living a healthier lifestyle than I do.

Never	Almost never	Seldom	Half the time	Usually	Almost always	Always
0	1	2	3	4	5	6

Outside forces—time, work, family—prevent me from living a healthier lifestyle.

Never	Almost never	Seldom	Half the time	Usually	Almost always	Always
0	1	2	3	4	5	6

Now, add up your score and see where you fall on the graph:

Healthy motivation	Inconsistent middle ground	Unhealthy motivation
⊢——sweet spot———	occasional wins, just as many losses———	harmful lifestyle——⊣
0———————10———	———20———————30——————40———	———50————————60

A few things:

- If you fall on the right half of the graph, you will have to push yourself through unhealthy motivations. Nothing will change unless you become comfortable pushing yourself.
- Your goal is to move to the left on this graph. That's it. Get better. Get healthier. Push yourself not toward perfection but toward *consistency*. As I tell my patients every day, the Holy Grail of fitness is not what workout you do, it's the consistency of doing something every day.
- It doesn't need to be any more complicated than that.

And if you need help pushing yourself? Good thing you're holding this book in your hands. Feel free to test yourself over time to see how your score improves as you make changes, even monthly if you like—but the key is being honest with your answers every time.

CHAPTER 4

Rescuing Your Motivation
from Bad Influences

Some people have that positive fitness motivation and keep it, others had it and lost it, while others are searching for it. We are always in flux. Positive intrinsic motivation turns to negative intrinsic motivation simply because we get older and our desires and priorities change. Positive extrinsic motivation turns to negative extrinsic motivation because influential people move in and out of our lives, we succumb to outside forces, or hard changes affect how we view ourselves and our lives.

What keeps people moving in the right direction? How do we evaluate the unique causes of our own motivation? Is this something we can fix and grow—or is it like your shoe size, you've got what you've got? This chapter will examine how motivation changes, a key part of maintaining a healthy lifestyle over days, months, and years.

What makes motivation easy? Well, think of a child in love with youth soccer, with venues, friends, parents, and a whole social structure around the activity. Proper motivation is built in—intrinsic *and* extrinsic. But throughout the decades of life, it becomes more and more challenging. I've seen the best results in families where everyone is active together and it's part of the fabric of their lives. I've also seen the opposite.

Meet Warren

Let me tell you about another patient of mine. We'll call him Warren. He's in his midsixties and very successful in the finance industry, so he's got intelligence and drive to spare. I've seen him repeatedly for lower back and hip pain. We work through it, and he has a hard time, but the bottom line is he keeps hurting himself because he's sixty pounds overweight.

Warren's kids come to my exercise classes, and they really want to see him lose that weight, so they try to help motivate him. I treat his orthopedic issues, but I also engage on lifestyle and change. Warren's weight is all belly, the visceral fat that's most dangerous, particularly for a guy his age. It's serious because unhealthy adults tend to become unhealthier older adults. Warren's inactivity, age, and visceral fat put him at immediate risk for type 2 diabetes, and while I'm no endocrinologist, I would bet that Warren is already among the millions of people with undiagnosed prediabetes and metabolic syndrome. He's going to age and become ill faster than someone the same age who maintains a healthy weight and lifestyle.

Warren—a smart, driven guy—has all the knowledge, plus the resources to implement it. He *knows* he needs to lose the weight but can't (or won't). Why?

Blame the brain. I use that language cautiously, however, as I don't want you to think, "Oh, it's all my brain's fault. I can't help it." But understanding what's going on in your head is a big help in pushing back against unhealthy motivations.

CAN YOU CONTROL YOUR THOUGHTS, FEELINGS, AND ACTIONS?

Self-regulatory capacity is our ability to regulate our feelings and resulting actions. Some folks have higher capacity than others, and a lower capacity can really mess with our ability to make healthy choices.

A paper in *Organizational Behavior and Human Decision Processes* detailing five studies found that people with low self-regulatory capacities were more likely to engage in "defensive information processing," which basically means they'll claim any negative feedback or criticisms are BS and refuse to make better choices or improvements based on that information.[1] Folks in the study who were already prone to self-improvement had no issues.

An example of someone's own biases holding them back. If you're able to have an open mind and be honest with yourself about your lifestyle, you're ahead of most people who resist change.

#1 on "the Big List"

1. Biases 2. Perception 3. Incentives 4. Knowledge 5. Curiosity 6. Self-esteem 7. Self-efficacy 8. Control 9. Community 10. (It's a secret!)

Recognizing Our Biases

It's easy just to say our brains have two conflicting hemispheres, the logical brain fighting the emotional brain. Psychologists call the logical side the reflective brain, or System 1, and the emotional side the automatic brain, System 2. So, when you make a bad choice too quickly, "Hey, it was just my emotional brain messing me up, right?"

Okay, but how does that help? It's true, but only part of the story. So many other things go into processing information, forming ideas, reaching conclusions, and executing ideas.

We touched on this in the last chapter, so let's really get into it: Some of our biggest mental blocks come from cognitive biases (also known as *heuristics*). And let me tell you, there are lots and lots of biases. A sampling:

Confirmation bias: We consider only information that confirms our existing beliefs. This is a big one and incredibly common. We'll revisit this in the upcoming belief section.

Naive realism bias: We think we see the world objectively and have no biases (one look at this list and you see how naive that thought really is).

Self-serving bias: When bad things happen to us, we blame external forces. When good things happen, it's a result of our own skill and effort.

Actor-observer bias, or fundamental attribution error: When a bad thing happens to us, we blame external forces—not our fault! When bad things happen to other people, we blame their own failings or character—totally their own fault! Example: Your heart attack happened because your father had one at the same age; your neighbor's heart attack happened because he's overweight and lazy.

Arrival fallacy: We think that if we could just hit that one certain goal, we'd be happy—forever and ever. Ask anyone who's lost weight and gained it back if this sounds familiar.

Egocentric bias: We tend to overestimate our own worth, effort, or contributions to something (related to the Dunning-Kruger effect, or our tendency to overvalue our own skills and performance).

Anchoring bias: We put the highest value on the first piece of information we get, even though better info comes along later. (One place I see this a lot is people clinging to the notion that exercise is the key to weight loss. We used to think so, but research has proven pretty decisively that diet is the real key to losing weight. Exercise is a much better tool for overall health and fitness. It can be a helpful weight loss component, especially when maintaining weight you've dropped, but as they say, you can't outrun a lousy diet.)

Adjustment bias: A partner with anchoring bias. We start with the initial anchoring information and then make (incorrect) adjustments to that information to reach a conclusion that seems reasonable to us.

Optimism bias: We think we're less likely to experience a bad outcome than everyone else.

That's enough for now (we'll talk about other biases as we go). But I wanted to ask: *Do you see a common thread running through these biases?* I do. And it's revealing.

These particular biases can be used to reinforce one's ego. Think about it: Deep down where there's just honesty, most of us think of ourselves as smart (not just intelligent but wise) and, more important, correct. We have reached a place in our world based on our choices, and we want to think those were the right choices.

Some decisions made via these biases could come from the following motivations:

- A sense of specialness
- A place of superiority, morally and intellectually
- A need to see others as flawed

Interesting, right?

Now, I'm not making some scientific, absolute declaration here. I'm a physician, not a psychologist, so this is just an observation. But as you consider your motivational profile, think about your biases—and think objectively, analytically, not blindly.

- Why do you think the things you think? How did you come to your conclusions?
- Are your conclusions tied into you being right, or doing better than someone else, or downplaying your flaws?
- Are your conclusions doing you any good?
- How difficult is it for you to change your mind?

Ego can fuel biases and color your motivation even when you know your actions aren't healthy. The giveaway is when you start hearing rationalizations: "I don't exercise consistently, but I'm in better shape than most"; "I drink too much, but I'm okay because I'm in control"; "My parents lived into their eighties, and my lifestyle's healthier than theirs ever was"; "A lot of people say they don't have time, but I really truly don't have time."

It's hard to be objective about ourselves. But it's necessary and worth it.

WEIGHT BIAS IS REAL—AND IT AFFECTS HOW MUCH PEOPLE EXERCISE

People judging others by their weight is nothing new. But *internalized* weight bias—how people's own weight affects how they think about physical activity—can be debilitating and can hold people back from regular physical activity.

A 2021 study surveying nearly six hundred college students found that weight stigma, internalized weight bias, and concerns about appearance influenced their enjoyment of physical activity and contributed to avoiding it.[2]

Another study from the same year included fifty-nine middle-aged, overweight adults (average BMI 32) and found that those who had higher internalized weight bias experienced higher perceived exertion during a thirty-minute moderate-intensity treadmill session.[3] They found exercise to be harder and more unpleasant compared with those with low or no internalized weight bias.

The Other L Word

When you realize how much our society has fallen out of love with movement, it makes sense to ask: Are we all just lazy?

Yeah, let's talk about the other L word. It's a default judgment for a lot of us. If someone—and it's almost always someone *else*—appears out of shape or unhealthy or lethargic or unwilling to exercise regularly, what do we say? *Lazy.* Won't put in the work or the time.

Well, knee-jerk calling someone lazy is easy. Heck, you could also call the act of calling someone lazy to be lazy itself. Why? It requires no work or thought. Science has something to say about that.

We may be hardwired to be lazy, or at least to err on the side of inactivity. In one study, researchers looked at the brain scans of twenty-nine adults broken into two groups.[4] The first group was physically active. The second group was not but intended to become physically active. The researchers measured cortical activity when people deliberately avoided "sedentary behavior" and found higher rates of "conflict monitoring" and "inhibition" whether the person was physically active or not. Translation: The brain has to put in more effort "to counteract an attraction to sedentary activity"—that is, the brain finds it much easier to lie on the couch.

Some more info about the "lazy" among us. Researchers have a term called *need for cognition,* which is essentially a person's desire to think. People with a high need for cognition love brain teasers, puzzles, and working things out in their head. Some people embrace it, others not so much. A study in the *Journal of Health Psychology* found that folks with a higher need for cognition were less physically active.[5] The less intellectual folks exercised more.

Does that mean the thinkers among us are lazier? Or dumber? (Or does this study revive the old nerds-versus-jocks trope?) No. It simply means this: Knowledge and intelligence do not guarantee healthy decision-making.

In the days when our very survival was in question moment to moment, conserving energy and effort made sense. Today we've kept the tendencies but shed the need. An awful lot of us have to do battle with our brains to make healthy twenty-first-century choices.

Lazy Has an Even More Attractive Sibling

On that note, let's look at what may be the most widespread and powerful bias of all: *the path of least resistance.*

Everyone relates to this. On its most basic level, the path of least resistance is why people take the escalator instead of the stairs. And it sounds obvious: Why put forth any more effort than you need to?

Well, the path of least resistance (heck, some folks strive for the path of *no* resistance) leads us here: A pre-pandemic Global Wellness Institute report shows the wellness industry at $4.2 trillion annually around the world, growing twice as fast as the global economy since 2015. This includes a cool trillion for "personal care, beauty, and anti-aging."[6]

So we're spending and spending to make our path to a longer, youthful life less resistant. Meanwhile:

—Society isn't any leaner or more active than it was ten years ago.

—Poor health isn't just an older people's problem. The "wellness" of the avocado toast generation is a myth. A 2019 analysis of fifty-five million insured millennials (age twenty-one to thirty-six at the time) by BlueCross BlueShield showed that the group was less healthy than its Gen X predecessors were at the same age.[7]

—In the past few years, life expectancy in the United States has declined for the longest sustained period since World War I—and that's not all due to COVID.[8]

PILLS OVER PULL-UPS

Most people choose the path of least resistance when it comes to exercise—even though they want to be healthier. Consider:

$48.4 billion

U.S. dietary supplement market in 2021[9]

$35.3 billion

U.S. fitness, health, and gym club market in 2021[10]

We spend 37 percent more on vitamins and dietary supplements than we do on gym memberships. Perhaps this is the path of least resistance training?

Clearly we don't want to put forth any more effort than we need to—*but we really need to* because our lifestyle is making us poorer, making us unhealthier at younger ages, and killing us earlier.

The path of least resistance isn't just an "Oh, humans are lazy" phenomenon. It goes back to our brain wiring again—where we try to "counteract an attraction to sedentary activity." This is really important: Researchers call the perceived effort of something its "cost to act." The higher the cost, the higher the effort, which makes any cost to act a key influencer on our motivation.[11]

You'll see that *perception* is a real monster here. "Perceptual judgments," as researchers call them, drive bias. And bias drives motivation.

Here's one of the simplest examples of that: A 2024 study in the *International Journal of Behavioral Nutrition and Physical Activity* split exercisers into two groups.[12] One group focused on aspects that made the workouts more pleasurable for them. The other group did not. During the eight-week follow-up period after the trial, the workout-for-pleasure group had a 77 percent higher attendance rate at the gym than the others. And during the trial, the pleasure group enjoyed their activity more and had a higher rate of "remembered pleasure," meaning they perceived exercise to be a generally positive experience. Feels like common sense, right? One group perceives exercise positively, the other negatively. Which group will exercise more?

How do we get around our own brains? We have to analyze our cost to act and conclude: *Worth it!* And as you'll see, we can make the cost feel worth it through a combination of knowledge, belief, and emotion.

#2 on "the Big List"

1. Biases **2. Perception** 3. Incentives 4. Knowledge 5. Curiosity 6. Self-esteem 7. Self-efficacy 8. Control 9. Community 10. (It's a secret!)

Back to Warren

Cognitive bias runs strong in Warren—I suspect a combination of confirmation and optimism biases exacerbated by an unhealthy dose of taking the path of least resistance—so much so that pressure from his kids, advice from his physician, and even his own knowledge couldn't push him in the right direction. Consequently, we tried a different approach.

I wanted to engage other parts of his brain, reach him on an emotional level. He understands finance, and I think incentivizing behavior is one of the more interesting research areas (we'll talk more about the intersection of health and behavioral economics in a moment). So I engaged his financial brain and helped set him up with a prepaid personal trainer who comes to him at home. He also started basic intermittent fasting by establishing an eight-hour eating window, noon to 8 P.M.

The trainer is the key part here because Warren prepaid. He's got skin in the game. The finance guy wants a return on that investment. And the trainer comes to him, so a major cost to act—going to a gym—has been removed. This is how you use extrinsic motivation to push back against unreliable intrinsic motivation.

So far, it's worked. I can't report a miracle with Warren, but he's making slow progress and is sticking with it. Will he keep moving? I worry about him.

Healthy motivation can be that fleeting.

How to Manipulate Your "Cost to Act"

How do *you* get to a sense that exercise is "worth it"?

To continue with the price tag metaphor, how you perceive the worth of exercise can resemble how you browse at a car dealership. Sure, that model looks nice, and you say you've always wanted one, but you'd never actually pay up for it. Same with exercise: You say you want it and are willing to shell out for it, but at the moment of truth—when you have to start—you walk away.

That's why "cost to act" is a really useful measuring stick. It *reveals*. It takes into consideration all the unique things that define your particular motivations—your private biases, your deep-down wishes, your pride and shame, all the big and little things that add up to what you value most. Biases and perception are *huge* in this regard.

That's why behavioral economics—the study of how psychology intertwines with economic factors to affect our choices—is becoming an enlightening area of research when it comes to our health. Some major universities have even established research centers for behavioral economics and health (the University of Pennsylvania, for example, has its Center for Health Incentives and Behavioral Economics). When it comes to any healthy choice—food, fitness, sleep, and other critical things like taking medication properly—it all comes down to how we perceive our cost to act.

Incentives can help. Look at Warren. We found a way to manipulate his cost to act so he found it valuable enough to do the right thing.

Science is showing similar results. A 2021 *Nature* "megastudy" (thirty researchers from fifteen universities) recruited more than sixty-one thousand exercisers from a gym chain and devised fifty-four different interventions to encourage more exercise.[13] Forty-five percent of the plans worked, increasing gym visits 9 to 27 percent. The top-performing intervention? Offering rewards for returning to the gym after skipped workouts. That's how most people got their cost to act low enough that exercise became "worth it."

On pages 44 to 45 are some basic ways to change how you perceive your cost to act, all backed by recent research into behavioral economics and health.

Gamification. The term means adding game elements to nongame situations, and the easy way to think about it is to "make a game of" whatever you're doing. Example: In a *JAMA Internal Medicine* study, researchers recruited 602 overweight or obese adults and put them through a twenty-four-week fitness regimen.[14] The trick: Different gamification methods were used with different groups. Some included points scoring/deduction to move up achievement levels (competitive), a sponsor who cheer-led progress (supportive), or the formation of three-person teams (collaborative). The folks who received support, collaboration, and competition all had higher physical activity rates than the control group who received no gamification changes. And after the twenty-four weeks, all groups saw declines in exercise, but the folks who engaged in competition during the trial kept the highest activity levels.

Temptation bundling. That's a mouthful, but it basically means you "bundle" something you want to do with something you don't. A *Management Science* study took this idea to the gym, pairing a desirable activity (in this case, "tempting" audiobooks like *The Hunger Games* that the participants wanted to listen to) with exercise.[15] The trick: People had access to the audiobooks only while at the gym, so they were forced to exercise if they wanted to know what happened next in the book. The full-participation book folks visited the gym 51 percent more often than the control group who had no incentive. Also: 61 percent of participants actually *paid* for continued access to the audiobooks at the gym after the study was over (and kudos to *The Hunger Games* for being so irresistible).

Financial incentives. This is exactly what it sounds like: doing stuff for money. This is what we went for with Warren—he invests actual dollars to make his cost to act worthwhile to him. This works. A *Journal of the American Heart Association* study put a group of people with ischemic heart disease on a sixteen-week walking regimen.[16] The trick: If they got their steps in, they received $14 a day in a virtual account. If they missed, they lost $2. This is classic "loss aversion" bias at work, which says we feel the pain of financial loss more than we feel the pleasure of financial gain. This study put that to work with exercise. The folks who received the financial incentive in the study had higher overall step counts over the sixteen weeks—and the gains continued during an eight-week follow-up phase.

#3 on "the Big List"

1. Biases 2. Perception **3. Incentives** 4. Knowledge 5. Curiosity 6. Self-esteem
7. Self-efficacy 8. Control 9. Community 10. (It's a secret!)

You see where all this is going:

- If you, say, add competition to your exercise plan, you might put more into it and get more out of it.
- If you save your favorite podcast for your daily run or walk, you'll be less likely to skip it.
- If you make a bet with a friend on how many days in a row you have a workout, your desire to win money or bragging rights could keep you breaking a daily sweat.

See how all this works? Take simple steps to change how you perceive your cost to act.

That's how you beat your biases. That's how you work with your brain instead of against it.

Fall in Love All Over Again

If this really is a love story, we're just now figuring out what the heck happened in the relationship.

What happens when you fall out of love with something that was urgent and exciting when you were a child—something you never had to think about, something that always felt *right*?

Movement felt right. If you didn't move, you'd bust. Now, nothing feels the same.

Did it leave you? No. You left it.

Did it betray you? No. You looked elsewhere for satisfaction.

Did it demand too much? No. It gave back exactly what you put in.

We grew older, but I'm not so sure we grew wiser. As we aged, so did our brains. And our brains moved on. Our brains now push us in new directions, not always the healthiest directions.

We don't need to conserve energy for survival anymore. We need to *expend* it for survival. It's the twenty-first century, and the digital, handheld, superconvenient world is cushy and soft. If we don't fall back in love with movement, our life and health will suffer.

Think about this chapter you just read. What was it all about? *Perception.* How you think about certain things—in this case, what it takes for you to exercise regularly when your brain has other ideas. In a lot of ways, falling in love with movement requires the same ingredients of perception you need to fall in love with another person.

Movement needs to be attractive.

Movement needs to be fun.

Movement needs to make you feel good.

Movement needs to make you come back for more.

And movement can be all those things. Sometimes it gets harder to see those qualities, and our brains tell us to have a serious relationship with our couch instead. Couch is warm. Couch is cushy and sexy and hugs us and never, ever judges.

If all else fails, go with your mom's advice: Don't fall for the one who's bad for you.

PART TWO

The Ingredients of Healthy Motivation

CHAPTER 5

Knowledge

I start some of my lectures with a rock. Literally. I show the audience a rock, and I say, "Unless you've been living under one, you know that exercise is good for you."

Sure, most of us know that exercise—along with healthy diet and good sleep and managing stress and rocking it at work and nurturing relationships—is The Way to Go.

But knowing doesn't matter because most of us never use the knowledge.

Crazy, right? Especially since so few of us live under a rock. So let's talk about the first ingredient in healthy motivation: knowledge. We'll talk about the one talent you can develop that is the key to all knowledge—everything you need to know about everything you need to know. And let's go even further than *that*. I'll let you in on the one piece of knowledge that can totally unlock healthier motivation for you.

Shiny new tools in your psychological toolbox.

All you have to do is use them.

You Do Know You Have a Toolbox, Right?

Several years ago, a study came out about heart attack patients that stunned me. I'll preface this with some other research I've read: 20 to

30 percent of medical prescriptions are never filled, and nearly half of patients don't take medications for chronic diseases as they were prescribed.[1]

That sounds self-destructive on the surface. To be fair, not everyone can afford the medication prescribed, but that's a separate issue. A whole lot of people *can* afford it.

But let's talk about that heart attack study. Researchers from Rutgers looked at two groups of heart attack survivors. One group of 499 people were prescribed beta-blockers, and another 526 people were prescribed angiotensin-converting enzyme (ACE) inhibitors. Both drugs are common treatments for preventing a second heart attack after surviving the first and, if warranted, can be taken long term.[2]

So let's set the scene: You've had a heart attack, one of the most frightening and life-altering experiences a person can have. You almost died. Your doctor tells you one or both of these meds will go a long way toward preventing another heart attack. But you must take them long term.

Do you take the meds?

The people in the study took the meds—until they didn't. After thirty days, 6 percent of the beta-blocker people stopped. Seven percent of the ACE inhibitor folks also quit after a month. More and more dropped over time. After two years, half the people prescribed these drugs had stopped taking them.

Risky behavior, right? We're not talking about joining a gym on New Year's Day and falling off before March 1. We're talking about heart attack survivors given a shot at preventing a second attack.

We can't say that affordability was an issue here. All study participants had continuous medical insurance and prescription drug coverage over those two years, and both drugs cost folks $5 for a three-month mail-order supply or $5 for one month at a pharmacy.

Here's another bit of research that looks from a different angle but with similar results. A 2024 *BMJ* review covering 129 studies of nearly twenty-eight thousand people analyzed the effectiveness of behavioral interventions on exercise motivation—in this case, "motivational interviewing," where a medical professional engaged with a participant to encourage more physical activity.[3] In most cases, the participant had an existing health condition, and the purpose of the exercise intervention was to improve or maintain the condition. So think of it this way: The interviews were designed to help the patient with all three ingredients of healthy motivation, knowledge, emotion, and belief. What happened? Increases in total physical activity (the equivalent of 1,323 steps per day) and reductions in sedentary time (fifty-one minutes a day). But here's the nasty catch: The positive effects waned over time, and people stopped exercising, with zero evidence of increased physical activity after one year.

So these folks were given an advantage most people don't have—someone encouraging them to move more and offering them all the support they needed—and despite that, they didn't keep up with the healthy activity that could improve their existing health problem. They didn't use the tools that they had in their toolbox.

I tell you about these studies not so you'll sit in judgment of people stopping cheap and proven medical interventions. I tell you about them so you can see that motivation can push anyone, even those with serious health risks, to do the unhealthy thing—even when they know better.

More Tools Gathering Dust

Here's another good example of the fantastic potential of knowledge and the incredible failure of people to use it: Workplace wellness programs are a common benefit nowadays. Depending on company culture, this could mean simple initiatives like skin cancer screenings or a more holistic push for general well-being.

On paper, this is a fair trade-off. Employees receive wellness benefits, and the company has healthier, more productive employees. And both parties have lower out-of-pocket healthcare costs. Win-win.

It would be really, really hard to call these initiatives negative. But here's the thing: A *JAMA* study observed thirty-three thousand workers at BJ's Wholesale Club for eighteen months when the company launched an employee wellness initiative and found that, yeah, folks increased their knowledge about exercise and healthier habits. However, fewer than 10 percent started exercising, and only a few more tried to lose weight. None of their physical outcomes, like blood pressure and fasting glucose, improved. To boot, their health costs didn't budge. Knowledge didn't move the needle.[4]

Research has shown time and again that regular physical activity can help improve, prevent, or cure virtually any medical condition—particularly the most serious conditions like type 2 diabetes, heart disease, and some cancers (yes, this is my thing, so you'll hear me go on about it quite a bit).[5] On the basis of clinical research alone, it's one of the biggest reasons for the average person to move more. *And yet, so many people avoid regular physical activity.*

#4 on "the Big List"

1. Biases 2. Perception 3. Incentives **4. Knowledge** 5. Curiosity 6. Self-esteem 7. Self-efficacy 8. Control 9. Community 10. (It's a secret!)

So What's the Problem?

Why do we make choices against our own long-term well-being even when we know what the right choice is? Part of the issue is all those biases we talked about. We have beliefs. We identify them as "knowledge." They drive our motivations.

Those folks who stopped taking their heart attack meds? I suspect part of their problem is a bias called *availability heuristic.* This is a behavioral economics term that basically means you put a higher value on information that comes to your mind quickly and easily. You then use that information—choosing it over more accurate or valuable information—to determine the probability of a future event.

These folks, over time, get further and further out from that first heart attack. They feel better. They're living normally. And those pesky drugs, well . . . right now I feel good. Do I really need them? People are using the current "easy" information to make themselves comfortable with their chances of a second heart attack (they feel good, managing medication is a hassle—cost to act again!)—even though the more accurate, predictive information (the meds will keep them safer) is the most valuable.

Another bias is probably at work here: *fading affect bias,* where feelings associated with a negative event fade faster than those associated with a positive event. Generally, we're talking a fade over months and years, but studies have shown that fading affect bias can kick in *day one* after a negative experience.[6] The further the heart attack gets in the rearview, the less it affects patients' thinking. They begin to take health for granted again, like most people do.

We see this same behavior everywhere, every day.

Why do humans do the unhealthy thing when they know what the healthy thing is?

That's the question every health practitioner (heck, every parent, spouse, partner, sibling, and friend) has been asking whenever they see someone with the knowledge to help themselves refuse to do it.

The answer: *Knowledge isn't enough.*

Knowledge is a single ingredient that needs help from emotion, belief, and community to become transformative.

ONE MAN'S BREAKTHROUGH

A man I've known and worked with for some time (let's call him Trey) has figured some things out in this regard, and I asked him to tell his story in his own words. Here's what he says about being incapable of putting knowledge into action:

I've worked in health and fitness most of my career, so yeah, I have the knowledge to live a healthy and hopefully longer life. More knowledge than most, probably. But I never really followed through on that. Not to my potential at least. I always exercised in fits and starts, I'm overweight, and I gave about thirty-five years of my life to high-functioning alcoholism. That was the biggie. People wonder why otherwise smart people don't change their worst habits, or take up the dangerous habits to begin with. For me, alcohol was all around me my entire life. My parents drank, my older siblings drank, which meant my parents threw parties and my siblings threw their quickie keggers, and all I saw growing up was people older than me drinking. Aunts, uncles, cousins, all drank. I got to high school, started drinking. It made sense to me. It felt right. I drank heavier in college, basically became a professional-grade alcoholic. Totally functional. An expert in hangover management. And when I got into the workforce, every place I worked—every single place, even the so-called health-minded offices—had a deep culture of alcohol. One company would supply kegs for parties. It was all normalized. I drank my way through it. Now here's the thing: I knew what I was. When I was in my early twenties, I was alone one evening in my apartment and bought some beers and listened to tunes and just hung out with myself and at one point I went to the fridge for another beer and there was only one left. And I thought, Jesus, I just drank a twelve-pack of beer by myself in less than three hours—and I want to keep going. *I knew what I was, okay? I knew. But I kept going for thirty more years. Why? Because I was functional and comfortable. I knew I could work through the morning haze, I knew how much booze I needed, I knew not to be a drunken jerk, I knew all those things and that's how functional drunks do it. COVID changed the game a little, though. Working from home, no commute, I got worse. I couldn't find the OFF switch, and all the knowledge in the world couldn't stop me from crapping out. I had to quit drinking. And I did. Hardest thing I ever had to do, and I slipped twice. But I've been good for a long time now. Know why? I finally started using all the healthy knowledge I had, particularly about physical activity. The big-gest thing was adapting to a life without happy hour. Three P.M. every day the booze calls to me. I had to put up some kind of buffer between me and those end-of-day cravings. I did it with exercise. Each day around 4 P.M. I do some kind of workout. Usually running and strength training. And it works. The exercise snuffs out those cravings, and I can push through dinner and not drink at all and be fine. Before that I al-ways hated exercising at the end of the day. Now I love it. I need it. It keeps me sober, yeah, but I'm healthier and leaner now too. I knew all along what I needed to do; I just didn't do it because the drunken path was the path of least resistance. It's like my body was waiting all this time for my mind to finally "get it." Now I finally feel really good.*

Pitfalls Surround Knowledge

How much knowledge do you need?

This becomes a problem when people really do want to make a positive motivational change but have little or only basic knowledge of what to do next. These are the folks who want to cook healthier meals or join a gym but because they've never done it before have no idea where to start. Negative emotions take over—fear of being judged by others at the gym, fear of looking stupid for not knowing how to start, not wanting to ask for help.

Knowledge → emotions → belief. The lack of knowledge feeds the negative emotions and torpedoes any belief they may have had that "I can do this."

Knowledge also becomes problematic in the other direction when people think they know everything and willfully close their minds. All those biases take over because that's what biases do at their core— they shut your mind to new information and outside influence.

But sometimes the right piece of knowledge pushes you forward and hits a sweet spot with emotion and belief. It unlocks everything. I know this firsthand.

I want to show you how knowledge—or increased knowledge— can work for you.

How I Gave My Own Knowledge More Power

I come from a family of doctors. I mentioned my parents before. Two brothers and I are MDs, and another brother is a PhD/JD. So that's six Dr. Metzls.

For young Jordan, coming up short in the doctor department was the stuff of nightmares. I almost did.

Motivation to do physical things has never been a problem for me (some may say I'm *too* motivated to run and swim and bike, but that's for a different book). But once I hit adolescence, studying and staying motivated to study became torture. I had problems starting. I had problems concentrating. Which also meant I had problems finishing.

Let's just say I had problems.

In college, I had to work for it. I had to find creative ways to learn, even using music, songs, and mnemonics to help me understand and remember information. So how did I stay motivated to make it all happen?

I didn't know any of this back then, but with an understanding today of how motivation works, the source of my bullheaded push to become a physician was pretty simple: I already had my belief and emotional motivations in place. In fact, they were constant. Why? Because of one very important piece of knowledge I possessed: the process of becoming a doctor. Because of my family, I knew exactly what a person had to do to become an MD. I'd seen others take that path and could therefore see the path for myself, so it was very real to me.

Did that make the path inevitable? I was hoping so at the time, though given how hard school was, I could never be sure. But the knowledge I had about becoming a doctor helped me believe that I could become one. And *that* made me emotionally prepared to do what I had to do.

You have no idea how lucky that makes me. If Dad had been a plumber and Mom had been an accountant and my brothers had gone into the private sector in whatever roles they found, I would've been out there in the wilderness limping through my studies, knowing I wanted to be something but not sure what. Even if I'd said "doctor" from day one, I wouldn't have had the knowledge of that path. I can't predict how that alternate reality would've turned out.

With time I got better at the knowledge thing. Once I began to really understand how the body worked, particularly a well-exercised and intelligently fed body, I was fascinated and wanted to know more. My learnings were fuel: I could use the data in my own fitness and eating endeavors, but I could also pass on that info to my patients.

Knowledge works like fitness that way: The more I knew, the stronger I became.

That's how I want it to work for you.

The Real Power of Knowledge

Knowledge isn't just information. It's an ever-growing collection of tools you can use to smash your biases.

Knowledge, to me, becomes most useful when we feed our fire with it. We use it to lift our emotions and stoke our beliefs. Maybe it's because we read something new that convinces us to make a healthy change. Maybe it's because we saw something that reinforces the belief that our daily workout is really, really good for us—and maybe even better than we thought (confirmation bias working in our favor over here!).

That's what people miss, I think. Way too often we use knowledge to knock ourselves back because we know but aren't *doing* what we know—which, again, feeds the negative emotions and torpedoes the beliefs.

You and I both know things could go either way in any decision-making situation and that in health-related choices they'll go in the negative more often than the positive. Two sentences with identical beginnings and mixed endings:

I know exercise is good for me . . . and that's why I'm going for a run today.

I know exercise is good for me . . . but I just don't have time today.

Here's the thing: If you make that first, positive choice—when you know enough to believe "I can do this"—you systematically begin to accumulate more knowledge, which in turn feeds belief. Like so:

- First week of new and better choices = "I can do this."
- Second week of new and better choices = "I *am* doing this."
- Six weeks after new and better choices show real results = "Wow, I'm killing this!"

And so on. New knowledge fueling emotion and belief.

We *know* we have the power to make the right choice. And how we do that is becoming clearer here as we go.

When Killing a Cat Might Help

I mentioned earlier that I would show you one talent that is key to unlocking knowledge. It's not just a life skill, it's a lifelong skill. If you can cultivate it, you're ahead of most people out there.

Curiosity.

Curiosity is the path to more and more knowledge but also to understanding that knowledge. And more:

Curiosity opens your mind rather than closes it.

Curiosity invites critical thinking.

Above all, curiosity *motivates.*

#5 on "the Big List"

1. Biases 2. Perception 3. Incentives 4. Knowledge **5. Curiosity** 6. Self-esteem 7. Self-efficacy 8. Control 9. Community 10. (It's a secret!)

Psychology professor Jordan A. Litman, PhD, has studied curiosity in its many forms and defined it this way in "Interest and Deprivation Factors of Epistemic Curiosity": "the desire for knowledge that motivates individuals to learn new ideas, eliminate information gaps and solve intellectual problems."[7]

As I said before, I've been learning more and more about my medical specialty, and the more I learn, the more curious I get. The process feeds itself. If you can get curious about how movement affects your body on a cellular level to improve health and longevity, for example, or why cognitive biases affect positive decision-making, that can be helpful.

But let's get back to that bit about "curiosity motivates."

In a 2015 paper published in the journal *Neuron,* researchers Celeste Kidd and Benjamin Y. Hayden came up with a really strong outline of just how ingrained curiosity is in today's culture:[8]

Consider, though, how much of our time we spend seeking and consuming information, whether listening to the news or music, browsing the internet, reading books or magazines, watching TV, movies, and sports, or otherwise engaging in activities not directly related to eating, reproduction, and basic survival. Our insatiable demand for information drives much of the global economy and, on a micro-scale, motivates learning and drives patterns of foraging in animals. Its diminution is a symptom of depression, and its overexpression contributes to distractibility, a symptom of disorders such as attention-deficit/hyperactivity disorder. Curiosity is thought of as the noblest of human drives, and is just as often denigrated as dangerous (as in the expression "curiosity killed the cat").

In short: Curiosity is hunger. And if you get hungry for something, well, you're going to be motivated to satisfy that hunger. That's how we can weaponize curiosity for positive motivation and how it can drive negative motivation just as easily.

Over the years, researchers have defined several kinds of curiosity. Litman's definition on page 58 refers to "epistemic" curiosity, or curiosity relating specifically to knowledge. That has subtypes. "Induction" curiosity makes you want to learn new information and gain mastery. But "deprivation" curiosity puts you in an "unsatisfied need state," where you must know something, like what will happen next on your favorite show or the outcome of a Super Bowl you aren't able to watch in real time.

That deprivation curiosity can kick your butt.

A 2016 study in the *Journal of Experimental Psychology* found that a "curiosity-evoking event" that was not part of a larger activity participants were engaged in could reduce the enjoyment of that activity.[9] The study authors mention exercise specifically as a focused activity that could be diminished by "curiosity-evoking events" like texts, social media alerts, emails, phone calls, and other distractions. Sure, we'd prefer to be left alone to exercise, for example, but the pull of those distractions is "deprivation curiosity" at its worst.

And isn't it that type of curiosity that kills us cats every time these days? Our phones are handheld gateways to texts, doomscrolling, gossip, addictive news, and any other of a million distractions that add up to hours. No wonder people say they have no time to exercise. They're answering texts or posting photos to Instagram even when they do manage to get to the gym.

Let me paint a picture for you. If you observe my waiting room when we're busy, you'll see a bunch of people from all walks of life looking down at their phones. When a name is called, that person scrambles to sneak in a few more scrolls or struggles to shut off apps, their fingers swiping away at the screen as they slowly rise and pull their gaze away from the phone to come back to the exam rooms.

And if you think the cycle stops when the exam starts, sorry. I can't count how many times a patient's phone dings in a coat pocket or bag during an exam, and while they can't look at the text that just came in, I can tell they want to.

I wish I was exaggerating.

Weaponize Curiosity

It comes down to this: Will you use curiosity for good or evil in your life?

Stoke your hunger for more knowledge about health, fitness, exercise. You're smack in the middle of this book, so you already have a desire for this information. What else can you learn? Lots! Allow this hunger for more info about health drive you to better choices.

Even more fun: Turn your exercise time into curiosity time. I do this a lot. What will you think about on your walk or run? What will you solve while you're at the gym or sweating in your garage? Or focus on your exercises: How well will you perform today? What might unlock a better jump shot, or tennis serve, or hill sprint? All of these are playtime opportunities for positive curiosity. Physical exertion is a fantastic time for your brain to work in different ways.

Here's another strategy. A guy I know, call him Rob, was like most people and wasn't happy with how his body looked. He didn't deliberately say, "I'm going to weaponize my curiosity!" but that's what he did. He said, "I'd like to finally find out what I can really do," meaning physically. He was curious to see how fit he could become and how thoroughly he could transform his body. He wanted to *know*. So he used that curiosity to fuel a stretch of better eating and exercise. It worked for a time; then of course he started having the falloff most people tend to have, and he now has to remind himself of his curiosity and hit reset and re-engage. But he's also seen great results. As of this writing, he's down seventeen pounds and his resting heart rate is down to 48. He's not done. Curiosity is still his fuel.

And for the opposite, the negative form of curiosity? Take steps.

- When something sparks your curiosity *as a distraction,* think of it as your brain giving you a Google alert and hit Decline.
- If your phone pulls your focus away from physical activity or other healthy choices, put it on airplane mode while you work out. If being that disconnected makes you uncomfortable, focus on what you love about your exercise time: your steps, your reps, your music, your podcast or audiobook, or whatever it is that helps you stay on plan.

Bottom line, when "curiosity-evoking events" pull you away from positive activity, double down on the positive activity. If you wouldn't allow another human to prevent you from enjoying your healthy activity, don't allow your phone and your brain to do it either.

CHAPTER 6

Emotion

My friend Mirna Valerio, as she tells it, has always been "a big girl." Now, everyone knows what that means for a girl growing up. Back then, she needed something to give her some joy, so she started playing field hockey in high school for a coach who didn't care that she wasn't the fastest girl on the field or the slickest with the stick. The coach was happy she was out there. And that made Mirna happy. That motivated her to get better.

Mirna kept running and became a scholastic running coach. Today she is an advocate for all runners, but particularly for fellow runners of color. In 2018, she was a National Geographic Adventurer of the Year. Running has really taken her places.

For Mirna, emotion and motivation are a package deal. She uses emotion to fuel her running and her running to improve her emotions. "Running sets the emotional tone," she says. "After a health scare in 2008, running brought me back to a place of physical wellness, but especially emotional wellness."

Now she's also hooked on what she calls the "socioemotional part of running," running races that let her engage with like-minded people all on the same path, all pushing each other, all keeping each other smiling.

When I think about how much emotion ties into what motivates us, I often think of Mirna. She's an inspiration.

Which leads me to an unfortunate but necessary statement: *We're a deeply unhappy society.*

That's a bummer to say, and some may anecdotally dispute it, but the numbers don't lie. Life expectancy in the United States has fallen for several years going back to 2014, after rising for decades. There was a minuscule rise in 2020, but COVID-19 took care of that. Adolescent and midlife (ages twenty-five to sixty-four) mortality rates have risen as well. It's not that we're dying sooner that has me worried. It's what triggered the drop in life expectancy in the first place.

According to the study published in *JAMA,* the death rate increases were largely fueled by "drug overdoses, alcohol abuse, suicides, and a diverse list of organ system diseases," like liver problems.[1] There's more.

CNN and the Kaiser Family Foundation surveyed 2,004 U.S. adults in the summer of 2022.[2] The headline stat: 90 percent of those people believe the United States is in a "mental health crisis"—as in, the entire country is having one, not just one group of people. Nearly half of respondents said they or someone in their family had a severe mental health crisis requiring in-person treatment or a family member engaging in self-harm.

A 2020 study in *Alcoholism: Clinical and Experimental Research* analyzed death certificates over an eighteen-year period going back to 1999 and found that today's rate of alcohol-related deaths is double what it used to be.[3]

Suicide, drug use, and alcoholism all tie into the same thing: mental health. No surprise, then, that recent health insurance reports show a rise in depression treatment across all age groups, but teens in particular. An American Psychological Association study in the *Journal of Abnormal Psychology* found that depression, mood disorders, and suicide ideation have dramatically increased since 2005, particularly in the eighteen to twenty-five age group.[4] Given that so many people don't come forward for help, the numbers are no doubt higher.

Of course, these stats intertwine with our overall health statistics, which are awful.

And this, coupled with a story like Mirna's at the success end of the spectrum, gives us a big window into how deeply emotion dictates our actions.

"NATURE'S ANTIDEPRESSANT" IS REAL MEDICINE

Research has shown for quite some time that physical activity has a positive effect on depression symptoms, so much so that newer research suggests physicians should be prescribing physical activity for the condition, just as they would a drug.

A 2023 review of forty-one studies in the *British Journal of Sports Medicine* concluded that exercise is effective enough in fighting depression that it should be considered "an evidence-based treatment option."[5] The researchers recommended moderate-intensity aerobic exercise and exercise in groups.

How Do You Flip the Switch?

Meet Randi. She's a fifty-something mother of three daughters and came to see me some time back with an ankle fracture. Randi was like most people. She had been a busy mom for a long time, had no exercise routine, was overweight. But the ankle fracture was a final straw for her. She was tired of how she felt, tired of the lifestyle she was living, all of it. I did what I do and helped point her in the right direction.

Now, a lot of people are tired of how they're living and how they look and feel. But Randi decided to do something about it. As her ankle healed, she improved her diet and started working around the injury. Once she was back on her feet, she made exercise part of her daily life, both cardio and strength training. A year later she'd lost seventy-five pounds and was running 10Ks with two of her daughters.

Randi hit an emotional raw point: anger and sadness at her current state, having a broken ankle that might not have broken in the first place if she'd been an active person at a healthy weight. And she decided.

I'm doing this, this isn't a quick fix, this is the new me.

Everyone knows a Randi: a person who has transformed their life—lost a lot of weight or made permanent lifestyle changes or achieved some impressive fitness goal. And not only did they do it, but they kept on doing it. And of course, everyone knows someone (or a lot of someones) who gave it a shot, made it work for a while, but ultimately couldn't push through and wound up backsliding into the old ways. Maybe that was you?

What's the difference between someone who breaks through and someone who doesn't? Is one person superior to the other? No. Is one person stronger, emotionally and physically, than the other? Not necessarily. Is one person smarter than the other? IQ doesn't have much to do with it—both people are intelligent enough to recognize that change would be beneficial. Does one person have more information than the other? Nope, we've already established that the knowledge is out there for everyone to use (or ignore, in many cases).

So what's the big secret?

A person who applies all the knowledge and resources—and does the necessary work—to change his or her life has decided, *I'm doing this, this isn't a quick fix, this is the new me.* And that decision came from a place of serious emotional depth. Something reached this person on a level deep enough to flip a switch, pull a trigger, name your metaphor. That's the tipping point. Knowledge is just a tool you can use or ignore. But the motivation to use it—once and for all—comes from that emotionally driven moment that finally lets you believe "I can do this."

I'm doing this, this isn't a quick fix, this is the new me.

What pulls that emotional trigger? Well, when you think of people you know who changed their lives, see if any of these ring true:

- *You get a health reality check* like a prediabetes diagnosis, a bad blood test, a doctor's stern warning (hey, some folks listen to doctors!), or some other undeniable and ominous health signal.
- *You experience a terrifying health incident.* This is bigger than just a reality check (people can ignore those). Chest pains. Waking up with blurry vision. Nerve pain in your feet. Something that sets off alarms in your body and brain and says, *This is serious. I'd better listen up.*

- *A terrifying health incident happens to someone you love.* Dad dies of a thunderclap heart attack. Mom's hospitalized because she ignored diabetes symptoms. A sibling gets a cancer diagnosis. Your best friend suddenly has liver problems.
- *Your body fails an unexpected fitness test.* You have to make some sudden movement to avoid danger, or sprint to catch a plane, or climb stairs to the nosebleed seats at a football game, and you stop to catch your breath, realizing that you're more out of shape than you ever dreamed (maybe like Randi, you fracture your ankle).
- *You see a picture or video of yourself* and wonder, *How did *that* happen?*
- *Your kids trigger the revelation.* Maybe you can't run around with them, or they make an innocent comment about you in public about your body or all the cookies you like to eat. Or maybe you just realize, like a lot of parents, that if you stay on the road you're on, your life with them might not be as long as you thought.
- *You're happy on the outside but truly sad on the inside* about your physical condition and lifestyle. And you're sick of sad.

That's just a sampling. In theory, it could be anything—a person's trigger is as unique as their DNA. But something happens that touches them at the deepest level, and they have what alcoholics call a moment of clarity. It shakes them. Others have described it as "finding your 'why,'" or your true reason for doing something. The intrinsic motivation within shifts to the positive.

And just like that: change.

TRANSFORMING TRAGEDY INTO SOMETHING BETTER

My friend Jane is a terrific example of experiencing a seismic motivational shift that was spurred by sudden tragedy. Sometimes that's what it takes, but the outcome here is unquestionably positive. I'll let her tell it:

One Monday morning a couple months ago, I got news that a high school friend had committed suicide. We hadn't been close for some years, but this was shocking and brutal news. Mostly because, well, to put it bluntly, suicide just did not seem like her at all. I'd known she'd had some depression battles on and off for years but never knew it was that serious. She took her life with a gun she went out and bought for the occasion, and that was just . . . inconceivable. To know that this girl I knew for so long went to those lengths and made that final choice so deliberately. So that Monday I was shaken, to say the least. Late in the day I went out for a run to clear my head. It was autumn, a really nice day. And while I was thinking of my friend, I also had a really powerful thought: I get to do this. I get to be out running in the sunshine. It's a fantastic privilege. A gift. Now maybe that sounds a little obvious or even precious, but it was one of the most complete and sincere thoughts I'd ever had. I mean, we all come up with things like that now and then, and a lot of times they're performative. This was different. It hit harder. And every workout since, I say the same thing to myself. I get to do this. I say it in the morning sometimes too. I get to do this. Well, now it's been more than a year since my friend died, and the man- tra still lands for me. I thought it would fade, but it hasn't. I appreciate my luck now. I get to do this.

What happens if you don't have one of those situations to help you out? How do you find your personal trigger? If no real trigger exists, can you . . . create one?

Our best clichés were made for times like this: Take a look in the mirror, look deep into your soul, call time out, throw a flag, take a deep breath, hit pause, hit reset, reboot, and on and on.

I think just reading a book like this means you've already made your choice to change for the better. Truth is, you don't need a reason to make a healthy change.

If you want it, you can have it.

Emotions and Money

Emotions work in other ways too. Think about what you've already read about perception.

You see or experience something → you perceive it a certain way → you have an emotional response.
   AND THEN
Your emotional response affects your belief →
You become motivated in a certain direction, good or bad.

A person's weight can be one of the most emotionally fraught subjects for that person, particularly if they're heavy and carrying psychological weight along with it. If you have an honest conversation with this person, most likely, yes, they would love to be able to lose that weight and be healthier. But their belief that they can—their self-efficacy—has been destroyed by any number of experiences from upbringing to low self-esteem (we'll talk about this in a moment).

Emotions can be manipulated, however. Sometimes instantly.

How? A lot of ways, but let's just talk about one big one. Hold out your hand, and I'll put $1,000 in it. It's all yours. Ten $100 bills.

Feel better? Yeah. Money can get your attention quickly. An instant emotional game changer. Money's funny that way.

Researchers have been studying how incentives affect human behavior for years now and have shown pretty conclusively that certain, um, *bonuses* can change your mood and shift your motivations. We talked about "cost to act" and the behavioral economic link between incentives and health. Take the money example. Body weight and net worth can be deeply intertwined, and research shows that the more weight you carry, the less money you'll have.

How much cash are we talking about? Researchers have become more successful at pricing out obesity. A 2017 study from Johns Hopkins University found that an adult who loses weight can add thousands—in some cases, *many* thousands—to their net worth through cost savings on healthcare and gains in career productivity. The study estimates that a twenty-year-old with obesity who drops to a healthy weight can swing $28,000 in their favor. For a fifty-year-old, it's more than $36,000.[6]

Another study from Ohio State University revealed this price tag: $226 of wealth lost for each pound of extra weight gained, or $1,900 of wealth lost for every point of body mass index (BMI) gained. By this math, if you're fifty pounds overweight, you could be cheating yourself out of $11,000.[7]

This is net worth gained over time from being healthier, being a better worker who can earn more and not being discriminated against on account of one's weight. (And let's not forget that many social determinants of health are rooted in economic realities for many people who don't have easy access to recreational spaces, fitness equipment and education, and spare time away from long, low-paying work hours.)

So . . . after reading that, did you at least consider the benefits of reaching a healthy weight? Staying there? Maybe starting to move with purpose every day and eat more intelligently? Behavioral economics, man. Money motivates us, and it all ties right into health.

Now, money isn't *entirely* the point of this bit. The real point: Look what happens when you find something that takes your emotions in one direction or the other. Looking at obesity, sedentary lifestyle, and other health issues through different lenses like this can be a powerful way to shift your emotional response (which, granted, is usually negative when talking about weight) and change your thinking.

For example: When you think about all those thousands of dollars—and how your weight could be affecting your net worth—think about your overweight as losing you money rather than weight loss giving you a chance to gain money. A 2016 study in the *Annals of Internal Medicine* found that among overweight adults, financial incentives for physical activity were most effective when framed in terms of monetary loss.[8] Someone takes money out of your hand, that stings. That was my approach with my patient Warren. He understood that sting.

And how about this: What if you thought of excess weight as a physical form of credit card debt? You rack up the calories today, you carry the burden for years, and eventually you're gonna pay.

Or this, which is more positive: What if you thought of every healthy thing you do as a small deposit in your body's 401(k) plan? The health you establish and invest in today will pay all those dividends years down the line.

Now, think of all the things that affect your emotions.

And in turn, your emotional state is affecting your motivational state. Every day.

Remember Mirna, a woman who has pushed through many obstacles in her life—all with a running head start: "Running sets the emotional tone."

Whether you're talking about mental health or money or losing weight or simply finding your smile, it all begins by rewarding yourself with daily movement.

The Untapped Power of Perception

When I think of how perception (#2 on the Big List!) drives our emotions—for good and bad—I think of my friend John Young. John has dwarfism, which brings immediate preconceptions. People who see John's stature without knowing his character perceive him a certain way. John had his own perceptions of himself and his potential as he grew up. He was always told, and subsequently thought, that he should never expect much from himself physically.

Doctors told him not to run because he had spinal stenosis as a result of his dwarfism. His perception of who and what he was limited his life and health, particularly as he got older.

In his early forties, he was overweight and diagnosed with sleep apnea. That meant a CPAP machine at night. And that was enough for John.

He started swimming. Riding his wife's bike. And yes, against doctor's advice, running. He stuck with it. His fitness and weight improved, of course. But he needed something else, an element that had always been missing: physical achievement beyond simple daily workouts.

In 2009, he signed up for a sprint triathlon (*sprint* is code for "brief"—a fraction of the full Ironman experience). And that's where the magic happened. At the end of the race, as he crossed the finish line with a huge smile on his face, his young son—who also has dwarfism—approached.

"Why are you smiling, Daddy? Did you win?"

"No," John replied. "In fact, I think I came in last." (He did.)

"Then why are you smiling?"

"Because I did it," he replied.

As John says today: "That race and all the races I've run since have totally transformed my own perception of what I can do. I opened the eyes of myself and a lot of people that running and dwarfism isn't terrible. And my son is now in school and runs cross country, plays ultimate Frisbee. He's shorter and slower than everyone else, but he knows he can do it."

John is now a fixture in the New York Triathlon—never misses a year—and to me is the ultimate example of the power of perception.

How to See the World (and Yourself) Differently

When you hear people like me talk about "changing your thinking" or "retraining your brain" or some other catchphrase to describe positive shifts in behavior, understand that the force supplying that push to proper motivation comes from perception, something we've been talking about a lot.

Example: A 2023 study of more than 1,600 people in the journal *Emotion* found that folks make "emotion judgments" in consistent ways.[9] Those who experience something and then judge their emotions to have been positive tend to have better mental health, while the people who judge their emotions to have been negative aren't as psychologically healthy.

Perception drives emotional response. And that very word—*perception*—implies that what you're seeing/feeling/tasting may not be what you're really seeing/feeling/tasting. You're just processing and reacting to your perception of the thing. And that can be powerful.

Example: What's one of the biggest problems for people who start an exercise program? Sticking to it. The Holy Grail is compliance, remember? Compliance/adherence (or lack thereof) is the biggest reason society remains sedentary and unhealthy. People start—and stop.

The surface excuses run along the lines of *I don't have time, I don't like it, exercise is boring, I'm unmotivated,* and you know the rest by heart. But the real reason? Negative perceptions.

A *Frontiers in Psychology* study looked at the underlying emotional factors that drove exercise adherence—what kept people coming back every day for a good sweat—and here's what they found:[10]

- *Perceived competence,* aka, Do I suck at my chosen activity? That's the fear factor, not wanting to look foolish in front of others or to feel inept while practicing alone. Meanwhile, the only way to get better is to keep doing it.
- *Perceived social interaction.* Yup, the ol' community factor. Am I comfortable around others doing this activity? Am I accepted? Am I forging bonds?
- *Perceived enjoyment* of exercise when compared to work and other leisure activities. Are we having fun yet?
- *Perceived physical exertion.* Negative emotions tend to make people perceive exercise to be harder. Positive emotions tend to make people feel *I'm really killing it.* Working hard at something is satisfying, isn't it?

Researchers have a name for our actions in this regard: "perceptual decisions" or "perceptual judgments."

And guess what? One of the most powerful ways perception can be applied is through a cascade effect of better choices and more fun and more engagement with others in healthy ways until one day you wake up feeling pretty good and you realize that you've altered how you perceive *yourself.*

I'm doing this, this isn't a quick fix, this is the new me.

That's what John did. That's where belief comes from. That's ground zero for "I can do this."

Can You Really Change Self-Esteem?

Talk about a subject fraught with emotion: self-esteem. Just mention-ing the term can push a lot of buttons. How we feel about ourselves is *huge* when it comes to making healthy choices and can be a vicious circle: Lower self-esteem itself can motivate you to be unhealthy, with mindsets like "I'm not worthy of happiness, so I'm just going to eat and drink what I want." All this ties in with the mental health points I mentioned earlier. A lot of us just aren't in a good place in our minds, with self-esteem working behind the scenes to sabotage what positivity we try to introduce.

#6 on the Big List

1. Biases 2. Perception 3. Incentives 4. Knowledge 5. Curiosity **6. Self-esteem**
7. Self-efficacy 8. Control 9. Community 10. (It's a secret!)

Self-esteem is a powerful driver of emotion. And even though low self-esteem can dictate unhealthy behavior, simply doing some-thing healthy for yourself can slowly improve how you think about yourself—or, to use that magic word again, how you *perceive* yourself.

Self-esteem and healthy habits have been studied extensively for decades. Here's a simple one: Back in 1999 (Was that really more than twenty-five years ago?), a study in the *Journal of Nutrition Education* recruited 155 married couples and examined their diets.[11] The folks who ate the most fruits and vegetables (and the wives, interestingly enough, had the healthier diets by far) had the highest self-esteem.

Feeling bad about yourself, well, it also makes you feel bad liter-ally, with measurable impacts on your health. A 2019 study in *Health Psychology* surveyed nearly one thousand middle-aged adults and found interesting links between social support, self-esteem, and chronic inflammation.[12] The folks with higher self-esteem who "per-ceived" (there's that word again) better social support had lower levels of C-reactive protein, an inflammation marker in the blood linked to heart disease. This data points again to the health benefits of com-munity and social ties, but researchers said self-esteem was the "key variable" in the findings. How we feel about ourselves is critical to healthy outcomes.

There's more. Research shows more and more how our habits—the healthy or unhealthy choices we make daily—determine who we think we are. In 2019, a *Frontiers in Psychology* paper detailed the results of two studies.[13] Each was designed to test the idea that our habits make us who we are. Researchers found that those folks who linked their habits to their identities the most had the higher self-esteem and were "striving towards an ideal self." Put more simply: What you do determines who you are. Positive habits lead to a more positive identity.

It also may be no surprise—and all of us experience this on some level in school—that a lot of our self-esteem developed when we were kids. That's a big reason why middle and high school years can be horrible for so many people. Multiple researchers have studied self-esteem as it manifests in children. A 2021 study in *Psychology, Health, & Medicine* recruited more than six hundred Chilean schoolchildren right around age twelve and looked at how three common factors affected self-esteem: food habits, physical activity, and screen time.[14] In general, self-esteem had a "significant association" with health-related quality of life. The rest was not surprising. The kids who ate healthier and exercised more had higher self-esteem. The kids logging the most screen time had the lowest self-esteem.

What about that "happiest time of your life," college? An Israeli study of more than 1,500 university students looked at links between healthy behaviors and positive self- and body image and had similar results.[15] The kicker here: Exercise was related to higher self-esteem than eating healthier. The kids who moved regularly reported the highest self-esteem.

My personal take on self-esteem as a person and a physician? It's a raw emotional driver that, when nurtured, can lead directly to belief and self-efficacy: *I can do this.*

I often see that in my patients. As they get back to exercise, or adopt movement for the first time, or try to ramp up to another level, they all feel better about themselves afterward.

The math is not hard here. Self-esteem, at its core, is our emotional foundation. Feeding it with healthy habits—especially movement—leads to a cascade of benefits and fuels even more healthy habits.

And as the research suggests, the habits themselves begin to dictate our very identities.

MOVEMENT → PERCEPTION → EMOTION → SELF-ESTEEM → IDENTITY

I'm doing this, this isn't a quick fix, this is the new me.
This is big.

If the survey I mentioned is correct and the United States is indeed in a mental health crisis, that means we're also in a movement crisis. Emotional and mental health affect self-esteem, which affects healthy choices, which affect how much we move, which affects our self-esteem all over again.

I look at how exercise has affected people like John and Mirna and Randi, and I once again wonder what could be possible if all people embraced movement as they have.

If you want to perceive yourself in a new, better way, push toward healthier choices. Tie your shoes and go for a walk, then a slog, then a jog, then a run. Change who you hear in your head and who you see in the mirror.

CHAPTER 7

Belief

I have a big picture of myself hanging in my office waiting room.

It's a really nice shot of me, arms up, crossing the finish line of a half-Ironman triathlon in 2019.

Now, before you think I'm weird or some kind of serious ego case, that picture's there for a reason (my office is a motivation center, remember?).

My knees are sacred to me because I love running so much. Back in medical school, I blew out my right knee playing soccer for a club team at the University of Missouri. I didn't need a medical degree to know what I'd done. I felt the pop, dropped to the grass and writhed, and knew it right away. I had reconstructive surgery and went through months of rehab. And for the first time, this athlete knew what it felt like to lose part of his identity.

Couldn't run. Couldn't sweat. Couldn't get that joy I got so much from movement. Of course, I recovered. But I've always remembered how depressed I was when I couldn't move. Not just garden-variety blues. Depression. I felt other emotions too. I knew I needed some positivity, so I decided to motivate myself with goals. The first one was to just get moving again.

I also vowed that once I was mobile and cleared for full activity, I would run a marathon. It wouldn't happen right away, and I knew I'd have to work up to it and not reinjure myself, but I'd never run one before and it seemed a worthy challenge. So I did it. And I've run one (at least) every year since.

My limited medical knowledge (I was just a first-year med student) was enough to tell me I should eventually be able to return to athletic activity. Theoretically, at least. Nothing was guaranteed. But that knowledge gave me the belief that I would. And I used that knowledge and belief to heal my shredded emotions and say, "I'm doing a marathon."

Forty marathons and fourteen Ironman triathlons and dozens of other races later, my repaired knee has thousands of miles on it.

Then, in 2018, I tore my *left* ACL.

I was playing baseball, and as I made an ESPN "web gem" of a catch in right field, I felt something go in my left knee. Just like in med school, I knew what had happened as soon as I felt it.

Something you should know about me as a physician: My first priority with all my patients is to do everything I can to fix their problems without surgery. In sports medicine, to me, surgery should always be the last resort. Naturally, many cases are obvious surgical candidates, and you don't mess around with those diagnoses. But the majority of people I see respond to more conservative treatment. And I know a lot more today than I did when I was in med school.

The day after I tore my ACL, I wasn't laid up. I was in the gym working my leg muscles. I used my knowledge: I knew that strengthening the muscles that support my knee would improve my injury outcome whether I had surgery or not.

Of course, I didn't want surgery if I could avoid it. I went at this with the same mindset I did in med school—I wanted a fully functional knee, no limitations going forward. I wanted to run, bike, and swim into old age. But my case was different this time. I wasn't a kid anymore, so if surgery was the only way to get that function back, I would've done it. But ACL surgery is invasive and requires months and months of rehab.

Eventually, I built up my leg strength enough to compensate for the injured ligament and avoid surgery. I got back to running and biking, and eight months after that great catch (it wasn't worth it!), I finished that half-Ironman triathlon. As of this writing, I'm fully functional, no restrictions. (Disclaimer: I'm a sports medicine doctor working at a major sports medicine hospital in New York City full of other sports medicine doctors, and this was the best course of treatment for my particular injury. If you hurt your knee, please do the smart thing and see your own doctor, don't just say "I'll rehab it" because you read what I did here).

Finishing that half-Ironman was a huge deal for me. I proved a lot to myself. Motivation was not a problem: Knowledge, belief, and emotion were all squarely aligned. I sweated my rehab every day and got my desired outcome.

That's why I hung the photo in my office. When my patients are at their lowest, hobbled and in pain, I point to the photo and tell them my story. They see what's possible. As I said, most don't need surgery. What they need is time, proper rehab, and, yes, proper motivation. I say: "You'll be back to doing what you love. Right there is proof. I was worse off than you are. Just trust the process."

I use that photo to create belief.

"Expectations of Personal Efficacy Determine Whether Coping Behavior Will Be Initiated" and Other Simple Truths

Belief is not a trick term here. I'm not talking about religious or political belief, or the things you "think" might be true but that can't really be proven (sorry, Bigfoot fans). I'm talking about belief in yourself, in your own capabilities, in your own potential.

That's tricky for a lot of people. I know some folks just don't think all that much of themselves, or they harbor doubts about their physical abilities. That's how knowledge and emotion become so intricately tied up with belief: Even if you know what it takes to do something, you simply may not believe you can. So let's talk about it.

Psychologists have a term for this kind of belief: *self-efficacy*. Think of it as a fancy term for "I think I can." Psychologist Albert Bandura coined it in 1977, and the research started piling up.[1] It's pretty simple: The higher your self-efficacy—or belief you can accomplish something—the higher your chances of doing just that. A lot of things affect your self-efficacy.

Examples:

- I've never done this before.
- It's really hard.
- I have low self-esteem.
- No one else thinks I can.

As Bandura poetically stated: *It is hypothesized that expectations of personal efficacy determine whether coping behavior will be initiated, how much effort will be expended, and how long it will be sustained in the face of obstacles and aversive experiences.*

Put that in the context of regular physical activity, and it shakes out like this: *The more you believe you can make exercise a go-to daily activity, the more likely you'll start today, put more effort into it as you succeed, and keep it going long term even though it isn't easy.*

Bandura also published a book in 1995 called *Self-Efficacy in Changing Societies.*[2] The opening salvo in chapter 1 is a beauty and sums up something I wholly believe when it comes to belief, self-efficacy, and self-confidence: *People strive to exert control over events that affect their lives. By exerting influence in spheres over which they can command some control, they are better able to realize desired futures and to forestall undesired ones.*

Part of self-efficacy is belief that you can control your own fate. It really boils down to the expression "I've got this."

#7 and #8 on the Big List
1. Biases 2. Perception 3. Incentives 4. Knowledge 5. Curiosity 6. Self-esteem
7. Self-efficacy 8. Control 9. Community 10. (It's a secret!)

Researchers have had a field day over the years with this, and the results have been largely the same whether they're looking at, say, the academic performance of college kids or, closer to what we're talking about in this book, sports performance.[3]

Belief is such a huge ingredient in healthy motivation because it has such a huge influence on whether you'll even start something positive. Meanwhile, the things coming out of our knowledge and emotions—positive or negative—influence our belief.

> *Can I do this?* →
> *I know what I need to make this happen (knowledge).* →
> *I feel ready to do this (emotion).* →
> **Yes I can.**

> *Can I do this?* →
> *I know I should, but here are the reasons I probably won't.* →
> *I don't feel ready to do this.* →
> **No I can't.**

The simplicity of this is so plain that people feel the need to make it all so complex by weaving a long intertwining list of excuses why they can't do something. Know what I think? Some people see the simplicity of this and feel threatened by it, feel like, *There's no way I could be in the wrong here, it can't be that simple, there have to be more complicated reasons why I'm not doing what I should for myself.* So they invent the complexity to let themselves off the hook (remember what I said a while back about our internal biases being based on a need to feel superior or correct?). They sabotage their own belief that a simple thing like daily movement can be done. *It can't be simple. Because if it's so simple, what does that say about me not being able to do it?*

You can see this person's self-efficacy collapse in real time.

I said it before and I'll keep saying it: *Simple doesn't mean easy.* Regular physical activity is the healthiest gift you can give yourself. Cheap. Time-efficient. Proven. But you have to put forth effort to do it.

I believe you can move every day with purpose.

Do you?

I'm going to show you belief in action. I'm going to show you why, even if you don't think you can do something, you need to take two words to heart, right here, right now:

Try anyway.

CONTROL WHAT YOU CAN CONTROL

A 2021 study in *Experimental Physiology* examined how physicians prescribe exercise to patients.[4] The goal was to make exercise prescriptions as effective as possible when the baseline characteristics change from patient to patient. One size never fits all.

You can use some of this information to increase the effectiveness of your own exercise "prescriptions" when you choose your activities.

No Control	You Control
Age	Type of exercise
Genetics	Volume (sets, reps, mileage, times
Baseline fitness	per week)
Gender	Intensity (how hard you go)

Starting out, you are who you are. You can't change the things you don't control. So don't sweat them. But you do control all the rest: what you do, how much you do, and how hard you push. Focus on what you can control, and your movement will become tailor-made for what you can do—and how much you improve over time.

Shut Down Doubt

Doubt comes in many forms.

For my friend Anne, age fifty-one and a fellow New Yorker, it was the worst form: She doubted if she would live to see fifty.

Anne is the living embodiment of overcoming doubt and fear to *believe.*

ANNE'S STORY

In 2019 doctors thought I had a benign fibroid tumor, but I kept going to the ER because I was losing weight and vomiting. I was told, "Don't worry." I think I went for seven different opinions. They even did a bi-

opsy and said it was normal, less than 1 percent cancer risk. When they were going to remove the tumor, the initial surgeon said, "We won't know a hundred percent until we open you up, and if it looks suspicious during surgery, we'll call in an oncological surgeon."

And I thought, You know what? I think I want to go straight to the oncological surgeon. Thank God I did, because as soon as they looked at the MRI, they said it looked suspicious. I said, "Get it out." It was a cantaloupe-sized ovarian carcinosarcoma (OCS).

This is an aggressive, rare form of cancer that has a high risk of recurrence and death. By some miracle it hadn't metastasized.

I'll never forget meeting the oncologist. She looked at me and said, "I can't tell you your prognosis. You might be fine, or you could be filled with cancer within months."

Imagine someone saying, "You could be filled with cancer in months." Now that I've been in this particular part of the cancer world, I see obituaries for OCS every day. A woman not far from me, a friend of a friend, passed away in October 2023 from OCS. She was thirty-eight. Her cancer went from minor to stage 4—and advancing—within two months. This is what I'm dealing with, and so far, I'm lucky.

And I just remember the anxiety, the grief. After that, every little pain was like, oh my God, is that a metastasis in my knees? Is it in my bones?

Two and a half years later, August 2021, it came back. One little lung nodule. I went for video-assisted surgery and had a quick overnight stay. The surgeon said to me, "About an inch of the lower left lung was taken out. You won't miss it."

Then he said the important part: "You have no restrictions."

I'll never forget it; four days later I said, "I'm going to run a mile in Central Park." I ran and felt pretty good.

Now please understand. I'd been an athlete, and my diagnosis hit me really hard. I thought, I may never get to run again.

So I'm running and I will keep running. When I went for my follow-up with my surgeon, he nearly fell over in his chair. I was wearing my exercise gear, and I ran through the park over to Sloan to see him. He said, "I'm going to have to use you as a poster child."

I'm using exercise to get me through all of this. My motivation is to stay alive for as long as possible. Being in the best physical shape I can will help me withstand surgeries or systemic treatment better.

But there's more to it. I have to withstand whatever may come physically and emotionally. I believe fitness is physical and emotional strength. I mean, I have days when I have to coexist with grief and joy.

When I exercise, I feel great. I'm doing the NYC marathon next week. I'm dedicating miles to various sarcoma folks who haven't made it and raised $45,000 for Cycle for Survival. I dedicate a lot of the miles, but I also focus on folks who are currently in treatment, and then I focus on myself.

In that respect, the social aspect is huge. It's wonderful to be part of a community of other cancer survivors and folks who've had family members pass away from cancer who are dedicating their run to people they lost. It's an amazing energy. It's healing.

We can carry a lot with us when we run. I straddle a normal world where I'm working full-time, I'm in remission, and I'm in an online support group every day and reading very sad stories. It's important to reconnect with my strength. And I have a daughter who's now ten. I'm showing her, even in adversity, you can build resilience. I'm lucky I can do this.

But I will tell you, getting my tail out there and running helped me get back into normal life and get strong again. I mean, my recovery, compared to a lot of other people, was extremely quick. And even now I think, I've had a chunk of my lung removed, but I'm running today and I'm strong. I'm going to embrace that.

You can choose to make an effort. Sitting home depressed isn't going to help anyone. And for me, it's not an option. I'm going to live my life.

If Anne's story means anything, I think it's that belief is often a choice.

She chose to be a warrior. Makes that choice every day since her diagnosis, in fact. And that bridge between *I don't know if I can* to *I'm doing it anyway* comes down to making your choice, to the two words I used before:

Try anyway.

Strong words. What happens if you try? You could fail.

People hate that. Some live in mortal, crippling terror of failure. I don't have data to support this, but I believe there are lots of people out there who would rather not try than try and fail.

Standing back, not doing anything, keeps you safe from someone seeing you and saying, Well, not very athletic, is she? Really out of shape, isn't he?

I could tell you that other people aren't thinking about you as much as you think they are. But you won't believe me.

I could tell you that other people, even if they do think about you, are more likely to be supportive of your goals than not. But you won't believe me. (Granted, social media can be utterly toxic to people who post photos/videos of themselves or try to communicate something positive.)

Self-efficacy deflates when you allow doubt in your capabilities to creep in, when in a lot of cases it's just ignorance. You don't know what you're really capable of.

That's why you need to try anyway.

Let's talk about the worst that could happen.

The Art of Successful Failure

Belief comes from so many sources. Knowledge, of course. And emotions can create belief out of thin air. That's why belief, emotion, and knowledge are so intertwined. One is constantly affecting the others. They come together to form your mindset.

But setting aside the influence of knowledge and emotion, belief, once it's in place in a positive way ("I can do this"), becomes important because it's the seed of goals.

We'll talk a lot about goals in this part of the book. To me, goals walk hand in hand with belief because believing you can reach a certain goal is part of the bedrock of motivation. But goals can be tricky. They can fuel belief. They can also sabotage belief (more on that in a moment).

Goal-setting science goes back decades, particularly as it applies to business and employee performance. Yes, goals are still powerful when it comes to belief. Science shows that setting big goals is effective. Science shows setting small incremental goals is effective.

To me, the size of the goal isn't important when you're just starting out. I'm interested in the progression in which you arrive at the idea of the first goal, and a healthy progression looks like this:

Your current state → *A triggering event (instant or gradual)*
    alters some combination of knowledge/belief/emotion →
    You finally say, honestly, "I can do this" → *You set a goal* →
    You begin

(Note: In this flow, the phrase "I can do this" can also be something like "I need to do this" or even "Something has to change." You simply believe you must do something different now.)

What happens next? Well, maybe you hit the goal, maybe you don't. For my money, just moving in an honest way through this progression is a *massive* win.

"Wait," you say. "I've done that before and started a diet/exercise/career/relationship/financial plan, and I totally failed. How's that a win?"

Failure can be a big win. Don't believe me? Then you may have never heard the expression *failing to success.*

Here are some hypothetical but very realistic "fails":

- I wanted to run a marathon, but on race day I felt horrible and had to bail at mile 16. It was just too hard.
- I wanted to lose fifty pounds in twelve months. I only lost eighteen.
- I wanted to earn $10,000 more this year and barely hit half of that.

You could make up a hundred of these, but look at what's going on. Sure, each person came up short on their goals—in some cases, way short. But what if I told you the following:

- That first person ran *sixteen miles* in one shot. That's light-years further than the majority of society can run, and they're also now incredibly fit, to boot.

- The second person lost eighteen pounds. How many people vow to lose even ten pounds and never do?
- The third person banked an extra five grand. Who doesn't want to bank an extra $5K?

Hidden within every single one of these "failures" was a success worth celebrating. They didn't hit goals, but they *hit,* period.

Guess what we're talking about again? Perception.

The lesson: Perceived failure can shake your belief, deflate emotion, and weaken knowledge. But that's perception only. Objective analysis clearly shows positive results in each case. Set another goal, and hope you fail even more successfully next time.

How to Assign Value to Your Choices

Belief is also tied to what you value. That can complicate things.

You already know I enjoy using behavioral economics to help us understand health research and outcomes. Corporate America (heck, corporate *everywhere*) has gotten into the wellness game more and more over the years. That, of course, means business-speak normally reserved for the financial sector is now applied by management to corporate wellness outcomes: return on investment (ROI, or how much financial gain does the program provide) versus value on investment (VOI, how much financial and intangible value does the program provide, like improved morale and talent retention).

Now, remember all those biases folks have? Well, beliefs can create biases. That's where a lot of deep-rooted biases come from. But the belief I'm talking about here is the kind that can help push you in the right direction: *Can I do this? Will this strategy work? Will this tool help me succeed?*

Whenever you talk about doing any healthy activity, other people will always jump in with their preferred brand. They're dogmatic. Why? Because obviously it works for them, and their belief is now unshakable. They've crossed over: Having a belief that something will work leads to knowledge that something does work.

That's a good place to be. The key, especially for people starting out, is finding what works for you. Wellness, or working toward it, is incredibly individual.

Some people are total gym rats. Others prefer their basement Peloton.

Some people are vegan. Others do keto.

Some people hike and enjoy being in the woods, what the Japanese call shinrin-yoku, *"forest bathing." Others swear by CrossFit.*

That's where business-speak comes in. Value on investment (VOI) is a real test you can apply to any new activity.

Example: When you adopt some kind of healthy "thing"—a gym membership, a new meditation app, a nutrition supplement—you're betting you'll get a good payoff on what you put in. Except you invest time and effort as well as money.

That's how you evaluate what's real. Before you buy in, ask: *Is this worth my time, effort, and money?*

Remember, what you think is a good investment is subjective. Here's what I mean: Let's look at a recent "thing" in wellness, "personalized nutrition." You submit a DNA sample to a personalized nutrition company, and for a fee they analyze your genome and send back an eating plan crafted specifically for your genetic makeup.

A few years ago, Habit.com was one such company. They used to charge $299 for the initial service. Sounds cool so far. And their website offered success stories of people who improved their diets and lost weight.

But here's the thing. Right now, there's no scientific evidence that personalized nutrition, whether it comes from DNA or artificial intelligence or algorithms or science fiction, works. It may well work one day. But we're talking years (if not decades) to assemble enough clinical, replicated evidence that it's all it's cracked up to be. Maybe that's why Habit isn't offering that $299 package anymore.

For some people, that doesn't matter. They saw the new, shiny thing and paid the money and sent in the DNA. If they lost weight or improved their health, it was because they ate more nutritious foods and fewer foods containing salt, sugar, and unhealthy fats. Users lost weight because—wait for it—they ate healthier foods in healthier amounts.

That is *not* revolutionary. But for some people, a DNA test and personalized plan are incredibly revolutionary. To them, the price is worth it. And at the end of the day, they still accomplished something.

That's why VOI-based belief can be such a useful tool. You see an ad for personalized nutrition, it sounds wild, and you see others have had good results. You ask, "Is this worth my time, effort, and money?" Some people will sign up immediately, pay the $299, hand over their DNA to strangers, and eat better. Their answer is unequivocally *yes.*

Other people might reply, "Wait, I'm paying all this money and giving them all my personal data so they can tell me to eat my veggies? That's crazy. I can do that myself." And those people go on to improve their health. So their answer regarding their own course of action is unequivocally *yes.*

Imagine: Two very different beliefs based on VOI set two people on different paths that were both beneficial and *led to the exact same place.*

Asking the VOI question can help predict what will appeal to you on an emotional level and keep you making healthy choices. VOI self-adjusts for personal values, belief, and everything that makes you *you.*

There's a Chart for That

Patients ask me all the time if X, Y, or Z will help them. *Should I take supplements? Do I need a chiropractor? What about the new/cool/happening trendy thing?*

I can tell they maybe *want* to believe in whatever they're asking me, but there's skepticism, which is a good thing.

I have a chart in my office I point to that always sheds some light on what exactly they're asking me. My default answer is "Try anything you think might help. I'll guide you as much as I can. But some things are riskier than others, and some things have a better chance at helping you than others." I put all these "things" into categories based on scientific evidence:

Box #1 — Things that are scientifically validated and can help you (e.g., antibiotics, vaccines, statins)	Box #2 — Things that are scientifically validated and can hurt you and help you simultaneously (e.g., surgery, chemotherapy)
Box #3 — Things that aren't scientifically validated and can possibly help you (e.g., certain diet plans, Rolfing, nutritional supplements)	Box #4 — Things that aren't scientifically validated and can hurt you but have a small chance of helping you (e.g., cervical manipulation, stem cells)

Boxes 3 and 4 draw the most attention because that's where the too-good-to-be-true wellness promises reside. The stuff in these categories costs good money and is hyped to the rafters, but it might not be regulated, or might be heavily debated, or might have deeply devoted tribes around it—people who believe, even in the absence of scientific evidence, that something is good for them.

This can get very confusing. Some people want something to work for them even if it's not right for them. They want to believe it will make their journey easier. I'm not a fan of framing belief that way when it comes to keeping yourself pointed in the right motivational direction.

To me, healthy belief is "I can do this." If the new thing leads you to that conclusion, if it motivates you to put in the time and effort, and if you follow through, then you're golden.

CHAPTER 8

Community

experienced something interesting about ten years ago. It's not overselling to say it altered my entire approach to medicine and how it intersects with fitness and mindset.

These days, aside from doctoring, I have a second role as a fitness instructor. This happened totally by accident, but in retrospect, it also helped fuel my evolution in the exam room.

Back then, I noticed that my patients who were doing triathlons, despite much heavier training volume, were injured far less frequently than my patients who only ran. That seemed counterintuitive to me. Shouldn't the heavier training trigger more injuries, particularly overuse problems? As someone who did both sports, I wondered . . . *What's going on here?*

Was it how the triathletes ran, the type of training, or the way they were built? I came to understand it was probably a combination of all these factors. One point became clear, and it wasn't the presence of swimming and cycling in the equation: The subject of *strength* was much more popular with triathletes than with runners. The triathletes I knew and treated had strength training in their programs. Runners? Not so much.

Right around this time, I was also learning more and more about my field, about how our bodies work and how my own body responded to new and different forms of exercise. I tried a bunch of different things. When I discovered high-intensity total-body strength training, however, it was like a whole new world of health, fitness, and performance opened up.

Total-body training made everything better—not just my race times but how I felt day-to-day: stronger, healthier, more energetic, and with fewer aches and pains, especially in my joints. Why did I feel so good? The muscle I built helped support my joints and connective tissue and let me work longer and at a higher level. Total-body functional training also increased my dynamic flexibility, so my body simply moved better.

That's not the story, though. I was so won over by that style of training that I started prescribing strength workouts for my runner patients who hadn't tried them. They felt better, ran faster, and seemed to enjoy themselves. Then I thought: Let's get folks together to do this. I began teaching free classes on the weekends to help my patients and area athletes benefit from the same strength gains that had helped me succeed. I recognized that it was much more fun to do this kind of training in a group, so why not create one?

Not many MDs moonlight as group fitness instructors, but this was really one of the most apparent ways that exercise and medical practice began to merge for me. Once again, I saw a way to help more and more people maximize their movement and raise their quality of life.

Then a funny thing happened. As time went by, the free community classes (called "IronStrength" because I wanted to help people build injury-proof, high-performance bodies) got bigger. Twenty people became thirty, and so on. Soon, I would regularly see a hundred or more people at my outdoor Central Park classes. And it didn't get any better than August 2015, when I ran an IronStrength class for more than *a thousand people* on the deck of the aircraft carrier *Intrepid* under the Manhattan skyline on the Hudson River.

Throughout this evolution, technology has helped connect an ever-growing network of like-minded fitness enthusiasts via email newsletters and social media. Fast-forward to today: Together we've built a global community of more than fifty thousand people that helps athletes of all ages and levels build fitness and strength in unison.

We've hosted IronStrength workouts all over the world. Now we hold three one-thousand-person workouts on the *Intrepid* each year. The spectacle is amazing. As the program has grown, I'm ecstatic to see how well everyone has done. I get incredible notes, messages, and finish-line photos all the time. In addition to having fun, the stronger the community has become, the stronger the members have become, and the healthier we've *all* become. The most amazing part of this group is how its members have grown to support and care for each other. When we meet in the middle of New York City, we create a flash mob of sweat, smiles, and support.

Texts, email, and social media keep all of us connected and— here's the most important part—*involved.* When you feel involved in something, a genuine part of a force for good, it's incredible. You feel like you can do anything.

That's why I know, believe, and feel that *community* is the most powerful provider and enforcer of "I can do it" motivation. If mindset is where belief, knowledge, and emotion come together in your brain, community is where they come together in real life.

#9 on the Big List
1. Biases 2. Perception 3. Incentives 4. Knowledge 5. Curiosity 6. Self-esteem
7. Self-efficacy 8. Control **9. Community** 10. (It's a secret!)

Are You Contagious?

Emotional contagion is a helluva thing. It says that the more negative people we have around us, the more negative we'll be. And flip that: The more people we have positively boosting us, the more motivated we'll be to do well, and the harder we'll push when we exercise because we want to be right there in it with the rest of the group (a little competition doesn't hurt either). Exercise intensity is important and healthy and the essence of pushing mind and body. We'll get into more detail later, but just know that I'll always encourage people to go as hard as they're able.

Researchers have looked at the connection between community and health for decades. If we want to jump right into self-efficacy,

Albert Bandura suggested a serious link to social ties.[1] Specifically, other people could help build your belief that you can do something. This could be one person, like a friend or coach, or a group of people boosting you. Today this sounds like common sense, but it also serves notice that seeking out the support of others might be all you need to stay properly motivated.

People have been studying for a long time how emotional responses can travel through groups. Back in 2008, the *British Medical Journal* published a large study following nearly five thousand people for twenty years (1983 to 2003) as part of the now-famous Framingham Heart Study.[2]

They found something far more interesting than, say, a hundred people walking out of a Pixar movie with smiles on their faces. We're talking about happiness spreading across entire communities. The study found that a person's happiness can be positively affected across as many as three degrees of separation between subjects. That's your friend's other friends' friends.

The phenomenon was seen among spouses, offspring who lived a mile away, and next-door neighbors. But there's a catch: The effect seemed to fade over time and distance, meaning that as people became geographically separated and disconnected, the emotions subsided (remember, the span from 1983 to 2003 was pre–social media).

The researcher's conclusion: "People's happiness depends on the happiness of others with whom they're connected."

50%

Increased likelihood of survival for people with strong social connections compared with those who have weaker social connections. A large-scale review in *PLOS Medicine* examined 148 studies of 309,000 people with an average age of sixty-four. The results remained consistent over age, gender, health status, length of follow-up period, and cause of death.[3]

Remember Alice in the very first chapter? When her knee feels good, everyone in her life benefits. See how health ties us all together? It's the same in your life.

Connection is critical when talking about the power of community. And this goes beyond just happiness. The connection between social ties and positive physical health benefits is well established, and research continues to reveal more about the relationship. We already discussed one 2019 study in the self-esteem section where strong social ties coupled with high self-esteem led to lower levels of chronic inflammation in the body (C-reactive protein, specifically).[4]

There's more. Isolation can be brutal on physical health. One 2016 study review found that strong social relationships had beneficial, measurable physiological effects like lower inflammation levels. Isolation had an even harsher effect on participants' blood pressure than diabetes.[5]

Doctors know all about it: In 2017, "social isolation" was added as an official risk factor for dementia. Being alone can literally make you sick.

Let's also understand there's a difference between isolation and solitude. The latter can be therapeutic. An easy way to paint this picture: Imagine someone going for a long, solo Sunday morning run that's both invigorating and meditative, versus the same person on the same Sunday locked in their apartment feeling sorry for themselves that they had no plans the previous night.

Solitude can mean exercise, or reading, or creating, or meditation, or any number of nurturing activities. Again, science backs this up: A 2019 study from the University of California, Santa Cruz, found that adolescents who chose periods of solitude felt happier, more creative, and rejuvenated. The negative comes when solitude is *imposed,* whether by punishment or from social anxiety or lack of a social network.[6]

Data shows that loneliness in the United States is increasing, so much so that the surgeon general in 2023 released a special report titled *Our Epidemic of Loneliness and Isolation* that details the negative impact of being alone—higher rates of heart disease, stroke, dementia, depression, and premature death.[7] Another 2022 study in *Aging* suggests that the psychological factors of unhappiness and feeling alone can add 1.65 years to one's biological age.[8] Isolation affects multiple pathways—our biological processes, our psychological processes, and, the big one, our daily behavior.

Being part of a community (even if it's just a "community" of three people) isn't just about negating the toxic effects of social isolation. Acceptance into a group is powerful fuel for self-efficacy—supportive people can build your belief that you can get things done.

In my experience, the size of the community doesn't matter. And in the internet age, the location doesn't really matter either. Fitness professionals regularly run online "training groups" of people scattered across the globe who work simultaneously toward their goals. Peloton-style bikes and machines hook you up to trainers and groups while you sweat—basically allowing us to access healthy fitness motivation remotely. That's huge for exercise adherence. And very soon wearable tech will allow physicians to track their patients' movement, vitals, exercise intensity, and more, and it'll all go right into your medical chart. The "virtual" fitness experience can surround you with like-minded folks looking to live healthier.

Online or IRL, I bet you already have an idea where you can find some people to join up with:

- Local facilities like firehouses, libraries, community centers, and parks that host exercise classes, sports leagues, and outdoor activities—often for free.
- Personal referrals. Someone you know knows about a group of folks doing something cool. They can arrange an invite.
- Social media. Family, friends, and online groups all like to post about their fitness adventures, including sweaty post-workout photos. Engaging can be as simple as leaving a comment like "Wow, this looks great. I'd love to join something like this."
- Start your own.

Like deciding to exercise in the first place, finding a group means taking that first step.

Take something as simple as joining a few friends who all want to eat healthier and lose ten pounds. Just joining up indicates an aligned motivation based on belief: "I can do this." And you know you can do it because you'll have company, support, and kindred spirits the whole time. Your self-efficacy feeds from all the positive vibes. You continue to say, "I can do this," because you have a bunch of other people reminding you of that fact every day.

"I can do this" quickly evolves into "I am doing this."

If the first half of the book is about information, the second half is about action.

The next section in particular will help you take everything you just learned and apply it to make meaningful change in your mindset, your approach, and, yes, your motivation.

Even better, as you push to make those changes, you'll begin to see—if you haven't already—how much of what I just told you applies to your own experience. You'll recognize your tendencies, your blind spots, specific situations that repeat and trip you up.

In short, you'll know yourself a lot better—or perhaps realize you knew yourself already but are only now willing to be honest with yourself about your approach to health.

PART THREE

The Push Plan

CHAPTER 9

Preparing for the Push

We're about to talk about actual, real movement in the coming chapters. The goal of this section is to give you a framework in which to push yourself.

What is that framework? It's a collection of tools—a four-week plan, a create-your-own workout template, detailed (and dare I say inspirational) writing on foundational exercises, more than eighty other exercises shown in detail, and lots of science-backed advice on how to get the most out of it all. You will use these tools to learn how to push yourself, become comfortable pushing yourself, and in the end create new and better habits that will solidify healthier motivation.

Hopefully, at this point in the book, you're coming around to the idea that movement for good health is work that's worth doing.

There is no magical force that will lift you off the sofa and put your body in motion. You'll tap your own power to do it yourself.

The physical activity is work, and pushing yourself to do it daily is work.

It's simple work for sure, but not easy work. If it were easy, we wouldn't be here. So far, we've been talking about a lot of hypotheticals and the theory of motivation, but now it's time to move your butt. No manner of pep talks or research or knowing how good it is for you can take away the fact that you have to work to get the benefits of exercise.

Movement requires effort and can feel uncomfortable.

Effort can never be effortless.

Sure, all of this sounds obvious. But this is what keeps people from doing it, so we have to talk about it.

Discomfort. Sweat. Effort.

Commitment to consistency.

Pushing yourself every day.

Even when—especially when—you don't feel like it.

If you've had motivational issues and are just getting back into regular physical activity, the effort you'll have to put forward and the discomfort you'll feel will be right in your face every time—so much so that you'll instinctively focus on it and think about many variations on the phrase *This sucks*.

Does it? Maybe you think it does. Maybe you *perceive* it sucking. But even when you think it sucks, well—so what?

Just keep going and do what you need to do. You can take breaks, give yourself grace when you need to, but never fully step away from the push, from what you're really trying to do for yourself. Always step back in.

Skip a workout? Yeah, okay, but remember that skipping is why you came to this book in the first place. Because here's the thing, and you really can't get around it:

A skipped workout is usually associated with a negative emotion.

Something made you do the opposite. Okay, it happens; give yourself some grace. No hard feelings. But the more workouts you skip, the more negative emotions you'll feel. Push yourself and you won't miss. The coming chapters will help you do just that, answer the questions about *how do I* and *when should I*.

So you need to hear this right now: Be ready. Pushing yourself is work. Don't let the effort required stop you. Don't let discomfort stop you.

With each successful push to move, you will become more comfortable doing it.

And you may not believe me, but I'll say it anyway: The work will make you smile.

That's when you're hooked. So let's talk about what it takes to get there.

New, Better, Happier Habits

The science and strategies for forming new and better habits could fill a book. Or lots of books. And they do!

New, better habits are not automatic. That's why the first half of this book shows you what's cooking in your mind when it comes to motivation and the second half gives you the tools you need for learning how to push yourself. That's where good habits come from.

Let's ask the big habit question: How long does it take to form a new habit? For a long time, conventional wisdom said twenty-one days. Further science says it's longer, maybe weeks longer, maybe months longer. I don't think it's useful to get hung up on this answer because, in truth, *we're all different*.

It also depends on the task we're trying to habitualize. "Exercise for at least thirty minutes four times a week" may take a lot longer to become a habit than "Read for pleasure every night." In fact, for a lot of folks, the exercise habit never becomes a habit. That's why people need to push themselves at first—and maybe even for all time.

Motivation also helps determine how quickly something will become a habit. Motivated people will do what they are motivated to do, right?

That's why we're here—learning how motivation works so we can push ourselves into better habits in the end. So, let's focus on motivation. Here's how this can work for you right now: The tools in the second half of this book are there to help you build healthier motivation and, in the end, better habits. The four-week plan is just four weeks, which may not be enough time for you to make pushing yourself a habit you don't have to think about. Or maybe it will be. That's not predictable. What is predictable is what will happen if you follow the plan and continue after it's done. You will have pushed yourself into healthier motivations and activities.

As far as forming habits, I suggest reading the many terrific books on the subject. Gretchen Rubin's *Better Than Before*, B. J. Fogg's *Tiny Habits*, and James Clear's *Atomic Habits* are all excellent.

A Little Secret When You Need
a Motivational Boost

People latch on to whatever works for them. You should too.

A friend of mine, call him Dan, is like the vast majority of people out there: nice guy, shows up, does the right thing, and in general leads his life like a responsible human being. Dan is overweight and will probably never be super-lean or super-fit or even want to be those things. He's always had a hard time sticking with exercise—always starts, always eventually stops—and really is the poster child for losing the battle with the middle part.

But we were talking exercise a while back, and he seemed more chipper than usual. I asked him what was up.

"I figured something out," he said. "A little thing. And it sounds stupid, but it's been getting me to go to the gym almost every day for a while now."

He told me he'd read an interview with a certain female celebrity who happened to be one of his life crushes, and she had a one-liner in there that went something like "Nobody ever walked out of a gym feeling worse than when they walked in."

She was talking about how she motivated herself to work out when she wasn't into it. That stuck with him. So Dan did what everyone is told to do. He carved out a time in his day when the gym could be a set appointment, sacred time he wouldn't mess with. And on those days when he didn't feel like going? He remembered that quote and started anyway (maybe thinking that he was somehow impressing that woman psychically).

It's easy to say this is the silliest thing—a grown man jump-starting his health because of a quote from his favorite actress. Don't judge. We all have to find the little things that work especially for us, recognize them when they show up as if they were said or written or created just for our little brains.

This is Dan's thing, and it works for him. And here's a hint: It's not the quote or the person who said it. It's the sentiment within that quote that's legit—and even crucial.

Of course, there's science behind it.

Start First, Get Motivated Later

Psychologists call this kind of jump start *behavioral activation*. It's often used in cognitive behavioral therapy to help improve depression symptoms. In Dan's case, behavioral activation is a simple way to bypass the entire process of "changing" your motivation. Your brain's like "Nah, no gym today," and you know that's not the right choice, so you go to the gym despite how you feel, and you do that workout. That's autonomy. That's agency. You take action. But the motivational transformation occurs *after* you start the workout, when your brain's like "Ha, glad you did this, friend. I'm back on track now." And you have a great workout and a great rest of your day because you pushed through.

Let Dan tell you what happened to him when he inadvertently messed around with this: *The other day, even the quote didn't motivate me. So I forced myself to go for a . . . well, whatever the hell you wanna call it. I said, "Just go out the door. It's better than nothing." Started walking, then jogging. And I had some tunes and I was moving, but I didn't really enjoy it. I cut the run short and headed back home. But I felt a little better the longer I went. I got to the park right near my house, and now I'm sweating. And I'm like, yeah, don't need to go home just yet. I started doing some sprints on the path in the park. And it started feeling really good. So I wound up turning this nothing of a workout I forced myself to do into a full-blown sprint workout that was harder and longer than most of my workouts. I hate to admit it was awesome, but it was.*

And that's the point: Behavioral activation is a critical element of pushing yourself.

Your behavior *created* positive emotion and subsequent belief. If you've ever heard the expression "Mood follows action," that's the gist of it.

Basically, you have to get through the first ten minutes or so and you're good. Why is that so hard? Well, it goes back to getting that big tractor tire up and rolling—people hate the first part of the workout the most. A review of four studies of nearly three hundred people in *Health Psychology* found that "participants significantly underestimated how much they would enjoy exercise."[1] Researchers attribute this "forecasting bias" to people putting too much weight on the beginning of the workout before they're warm and moving. Once they got moving, their enjoyment increased.

You can't wait around for the perfect mood—or expect that one will ever arrive that day—so just do the thing and let the thing change your mood for you.

This strategy (like exercise) has been effective in treating depression, for one. Patients develop a variety of activities that improve their mood—maybe something they used to enjoy, maybe something new, including exercise—and do those things to alleviate their symptoms even when they aren't motivated to. A *PLOS One* review of twenty-six studies including more than 1,500 people found behavioral activation to be superior to treatments assigned to the control groups—which isn't a surprise—but it was also superior to prescribed medication.[2]

Another review of eight studies by Spanish researchers analyzed depression patients who also had substance abuse issues.[3] Three of the studies looked at smokers, two investigated opioid addiction, two covered alcohol/drug dependence, and one addressed crystal meth abuse. Behavioral activation showed positive results in seven of the eight studies, as well as improved depression symptoms in six studies.

The more you move, the more you'll like it

That was the finding of a study in *PLOS One* that observed sedentary young adults for six weeks.[4] One group did high-intensity interval training (HIIT), and another did moderate-intensity continual training (think steady-state jogging or brisk walking). The HIIT group's enjoyment increased over six weeks (and with increasing workloads!), while the MCT group's enjoyment remained constant or lower. Bottom line: You might find that workouts become more enjoyable the more intensity you add and the longer you do them consistently.

There's more: A 2021 study review in *BMC Psychology* found that younger people in particular *preferred* behavioral activation to help with their depression symptoms.[5] And another 2020 study of thirty-one sedentary, depressed people applied behavioral activation and exercise over twelve weeks and "all participants significantly improved." Better still: The folks who used more exercise than the others had "greater and faster declines in depression."[6] (The research of "nature's antidepressant" does indeed run deep.)

But wait, you say, I'm not depressed. And I say, that's good! My friend Dan isn't depressed either, nor is he a substance abuser beyond the extra IPA on a weeknight. But this kind of mood activation works for him because he *needs* it. The majority of people need it too.

And we need it most when we feel lousiest.

Feel like crap? Get moving.

Feel sad or angry? Get moving.

Feel burned out? Get moving.

Feel defeated? Get moving.

When negative emotions are on the table, movement can be your immediate response. If you adopt that mindset, you could find yourself exercising *more* than you planned.

I keep saying the Holy Grail for exercise is *compliance*. Or *adherence*. Those are the five-dollar words physicians use for showing up, sticking with it, forcing yourself, gutting it out, and whatever other phrase you might use for working up that sweat each day. Behavioral activation is the ideal tool for exercise compliance.

So even when you don't feel like it, slap on those shoes and head out the door or pick up a dumbbell or get on that bike and see what happens.

Best part: You'll probably only have to push yourself for a brief time. After that five- or ten-minute window of conscious pushing, your body will take over and your brain will relent. The activity will feel better, and soon feel good. You give your joints a chance to get warm, your muscles to work at capacity, your neurotransmitters to fire in happy ways. And when you're done? Celebrations and high-fives.

Stuck in the Middle Part

Now, let's talk about mile 21.

Actually, let's talk about mile 8 first.

So, you're running your first marathon. You trained by the book, but there's so much stress. You didn't sleep well last night because of the butterflies. You skimped on breakfast. You had nervous knots all morning leading up to the starting gun. All of it just sucking away energy. And when the starting gun went off? You were so fired up that you ran the first chunk of miles way faster than you're supposed to, and they felt easy.

But now you're at mile 8, and you suddenly don't feel so good. Yes, you trained, but you slept like garbage and blew through all that energy from nerves and tearing out of the gates too fast. And for the first time, the fatigue in your legs and lungs allows doubt to creep into your mind.

I don't know if I can do this.

You're at mile 8. You have 18.2 miles to go. Do you have 18 more in you? Yes, you probably do, but your brain isn't so sure right now. The rest of the race will feel like torture. Doubt feeds fear, fear feeds stress, stress sucks energy, and here comes more doubt.

Congratulations, you're smack dab in *the middle part*. The middle part is where your excitement from starting and achieving early results has worn off, and yet—the final goal is so, so far away that you stop thinking it's realistic. Or enjoyable. Or worth it.

The middle part sucks.

Here are some famous "middle parts":

- The part where you've been diligently saving money or paying down debt but don't have a better life yet
- The part where you've lost some weight but aren't at your goal yet
- The part where you've trained, learned, and expanded your career skill set but aren't a VP yet

There's no research to back up the following statement, but I'd bet good money that almost all people who have started something good for themselves and later stopped did so somewhere in the middle part.

They stopped because the early wins stopped. The novelty wore off. The effort became more obvious and less attractive. The small goals started feeling meaningless and the final goal remained far-off and there was nothing ahead but lots of hard work.

Your motivation shifts (and it's not even subtle). "I can do this" is suddenly and so easily replaced by "I don't know if I can do this" or even "I have no interest in doing this." Your brain is motivating you to bail. *All that resistance you pushed through to get here, and now fate has smiled upon you and provided an immediate path with no resistance: All you have to do is stop.*

And you stop. Because that's when everyone stops.

How do you stay properly motivated through the middle part when the gains have less meaning and the goal is still out of reach?

You have to push yourself.

Can You Act Like a Professional?

I hate how obvious this statement is: *If things get hard, you have to push yourself.*

Well, of course you do! Why even say it? Because something even more obvious is folks stopping in the middle part. And you're reading this book because you feel like you need help with it.

Why is it so hard for people to push themselves?

It's more than simply saying our intrinsic motivation has shifted, pushing us to less healthy choices. That's true, but *why?*

To make daily healthy choices, we must now live a life where words like *discipline* and *consistency* ring true for us—and not just once in a while. Discipline and consistency immediately invoke work and effort: doing things you know you should do because they're good for you, but you hate doing because you want to do other, more pleasurable things that aren't good for you.

My advice for starters: When it comes to physical activity, act like a professional.

The definition of a professional, if you take it literally, is someone paid for what they do: professional physician, professional athlete, professional accountant, and so on. But a not-totally-unwritten definition of a professional is someone who shows up and does the work even when they don't want to.

How do they do it? They push themselves when they need to. They're willing to push. They're comfortable doing it.

The problem with regular physical activity and healthy lifestyles? They are not a day job with a paycheck attached. At best, most people consider exercise a hobby or a chore.

It's easy to blow off those things. You have no intrinsic motivation anymore. It takes extended collective bargaining sessions between angels and devils on both shoulders to even lace up your sneakers.

Right now, I want to ease you into what it takes to consistently push yourself: understanding the moment you need to do it.

I created the following graphic for my previous book, *The Exercise Cure*, to illustrate how regular positive activity can set a cycle in motion that builds and builds in meaningful ways as you go around and around. I call it the "Exercycle." Start with "Do your workout today!" and follow the arrows to see how your life will change for the better— all from doing that single, first positive thing.

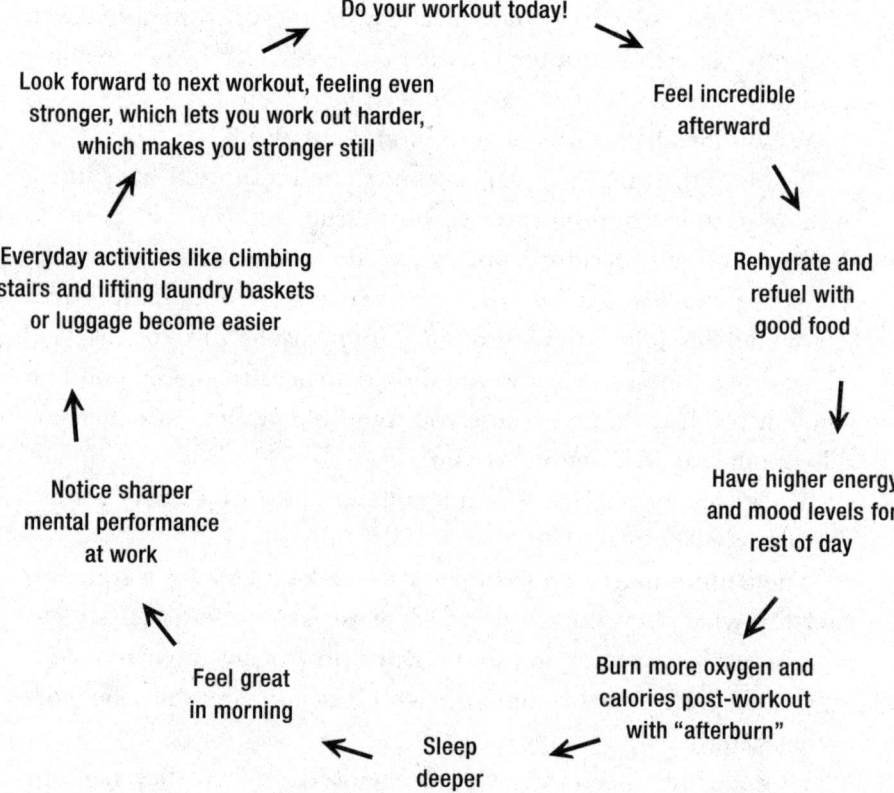

The more you do good things, the more you'll do good things. This graphic functions as a primer on what healthy motivation looks like in a self-perpetuating way. But where this graphic comes up short? It doesn't show the key vulnerable moments when a person needs to push because negative motivations fight for control.

Well, I'd like to introduce a new "exercycle," but it's not strictly about your workout. This one is smaller and simpler and is about all your activities, particularly the ones most affected by poor motivation.

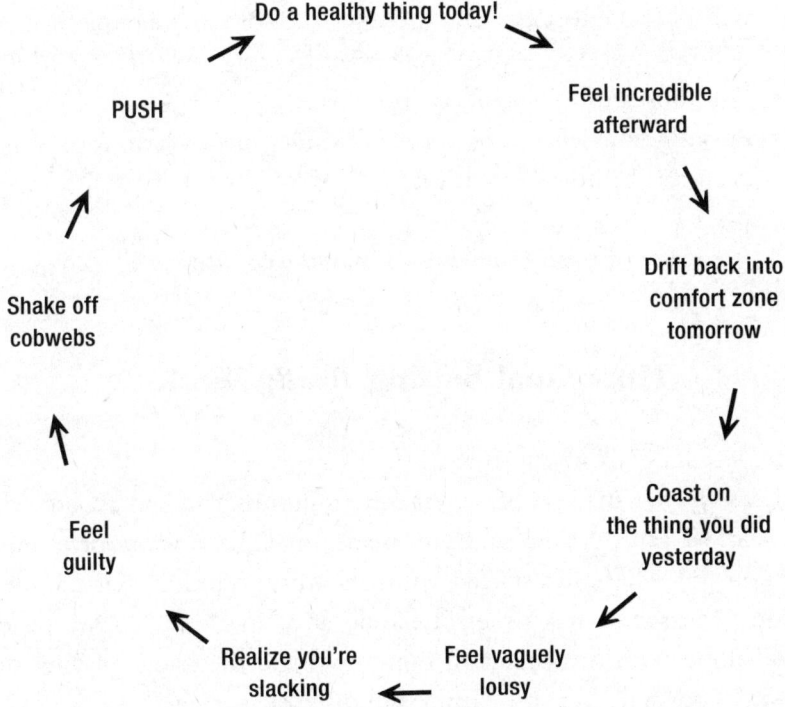

Do a healthy thing today!

PUSH

Feel incredible afterward

Shake off cobwebs

Drift back into comfort zone tomorrow

Feel guilty

Coast on the thing you did yesterday

Realize you're slacking

Feel vaguely lousy

Hint: You should not be waiting for the cobwebs to push yourself. See that third step? Drift back into your comfort zone? *That's* your warning bell. *That's* when you should push. Do that and the rest of this lousy cycle breaks apart, and you're left with "Do a healthy thing today! Feel incredible afterward, PUSH."

Keep following that pattern, and you're back to the original cycle where everything is positive.

That's the sticking point for so many people. People are uncomfortable pushing themselves. Or their behavior is inconsistent, pushing too much one day and too little the next. So, let's keep this really simple:

- Your goal each day is consistent positive movement in the direction you've chosen.
- Show up with consistency each day and you'll have that positive forward movement.
- Some days you'll have beautiful intrinsic motivation, and it will all feel effortless. Other days—and for some people it will be most days—you won't want to show up.
- You must push yourself on those days.
- Pushing yourself can be uncomfortable, so you have to become comfortable with it.

The beauty of this? There are so many ways you can.

How Goal Setting *Really* Works

Okay, *now* let's talk about mile 21.

Let's say you made it past your mile 8 slump: You had a Gatorade and said, "I can do this," and you made small goals for yourself just like you did when you started your marathon training. Eat the elephant. One stride at a time, one mile at a time. And "One more mile," along with the cheers of the crowd and the bands playing on the street corners, has you passing the mile 21 marker.

And you're hurtin'.

The doubts creep in harder this time because they seem so much more legit. You really may be out of gas. And twenty-one miles is nothing to sneeze at. You could stop. "One more mile" just feels meaningless now.

First, take a moment. Understand that even though it feels worse than ever, you're not in "the middle part" anymore. You're in the last 20 percent. You're almost there.

The small goals strategy that worked before and so clearly isn't working now needs to be adjusted. Making a basic pivot in your thinking could shift your perception. But what?

A 2017 Stanford study looked at goal setting in multiple areas like exercise, business reviews, and work-for-pay jobs. They found that while setting a large goal can be motivating but daunting and setting smaller goals to achieve the bigger one can be useful, the small goals ultimately sabotaged the participants.[7]

Why? Small goals were great in the early to midstages of each task (one more mile!) but became demotivating the closer people came to the end goal. The participants who adjusted their focus away from small increments and more toward the big goal as they came closer to it maintained their motivation.

Mile 21 is the time to think, not about mile 22, but about the whole damn race.

WHAT I TELL MY PATIENTS ABOUT GOALS

- First, set the goal. Almost every patient I see needs some kind of goal, sometimes healing based, sometimes rehab based, sometimes a get-better-than-you-were-before-your-injury goal.
- The goal can be big or small, but it really should scare you a bit. It should require real work and not be something you can roll out of bed and accomplish.
- Set a realistic but firm time frame.
- Set a realistic but firm plan.
- Secret sauce: Create or join a community that has a similar goal (in person or virtual).
- Launch.

Accept Your Vulnerability

If healthy motivation isn't your default setting, you need to accept your vulnerability. You're open to distraction, to temptation, to any number of things that could derail an otherwise healthy intention.

In other words, admit you're human.

Admit you need to put forth effort to succeed here.

Admit you need to push yourself to achieve consistency.

Part of intrinsic motivation is autonomy, a feeling of control over your fate (#8 on the Big List!). You have what's known as agency—a power to make your own choices and walk your own path.

That's not always easy. The path has side roads that lead to secret stashes and is also lined with sports bars, doughnut shops, and TVs tuned to your favorite channels in front of the cushiest sofas you've ever sunk into.

Push past them.

Just because you're vulnerable doesn't mean you're weak.

You have agency. You have autonomy. You have power.

CHAPTER 10

Your Exercise Prescription

Here's the fun part. Here's where we walk through all the fantastic and incredibly simple ways you will wake up your body.

I've long believed that physicians should be more involved in encouraging their patients to increase physical activity. Exercise is medicine, after all—cheap, plentiful medicine with no negative side effects and endless refills. I believe this so much that some of my colleagues and I now instruct medical students at several medical schools on how to prescribe exercise effectively. This is new. We're pushing for exercise to be treated equally as medicine the way blood pressure meds or antidepressants are treated (I use those two examples deliberately, given how well exercise can help improve your blood pressure and mental health).

This chapter is your exercise prescription.

We're going to talk about what you need.

We're going to talk about what to do.

We're going to talk about some of the BS surrounding exercise and how to disregard it.

Your first step . . .

Fill Your Exercise Prescription

When I prescribe exercise, I do so like any doctor prescribing any medication. I consider the unique medical situation of each patient and tailor the Rx accordingly. You and I are not face-to-face, obviously, so if you're dealing with a medical condition, whether acute or chronic, you really should see your doctor before trying anything physical. I know, I know, you hear that disclaimer a lot when it comes to exercise, but it's smart advice. Everyone should see their doctor at least once a year for a checkup anyway, more if managing a long-term condition, just so your physician has up-to-date information if your health changes. Your doctor may also be able to spot some underlying issue that might affect physical activity goals.

Another bit of advice before starting: If you're taking up exercise after a long layoff or you've never done it before, *go slow.* If you overdo it early on, you'll be doing the human body equivalent of stretching a frozen rubber band. Something will snap.

All that said, there really is only one rule you need to follow: **Keep it simple. Don't complicate any exercise situation until you're really ready to do so.**

Here's the super-top-secret magical long-term prescription formula:

DO SOMETHING. → ADJUST AS NEEDED.

What were you expecting? Of course, it doesn't look like much, but that's a good exercise program to a T. And here's another secret: You can stay on the "do something" phase of it as long as you want to before changing anything. The "do something" phase is more important, and you can see fantastic results simply by moving each day and challenging your body consistently.

Since we're keeping it simple, this is a good place to talk about the myth of complex workouts.

If you spend any time on social media, particularly a video-based platform like Instagram, you can find endless clips from trainers and fitness influencers doing complex moves you've never seen before. They may be fun to watch (we do appreciate movement, remember), but for the most part they're very advanced and maybe even question-able in what benefits they deliver. You should never feel compelled to do them.

An Important Word on How You Feel About Yourself

I'm a very gung-ho person. I constantly push myself physically and mentally, and I encourage my patients and IronStrength community members to push themselves. I've seen too many positive results from it to ever stop.

I find that being in a state where one wants to improve oneself isn't just healthy but vital. That's why this book is all about becoming comfortable with pushing yourself.

But I know very well that different people respond to different methods.

The idea of pushing yourself, of getting better, can be loaded with emotions positive and negative.

Here's what I want to be clear about:

When I say push yourself, I mean push yourself to move more so you can have better health and a longer healthspan.

I mean push yourself to move more so you feel physically better and are more physically able.

I do *not* mean push yourself so you look a certain way. Or so you can live up to a certain beauty or athletic standard. Or because you use exercise as a form of punishment for overeating.

Hey, I get it. Lots of people work out for exactly those reasons. Vanity motivates, and if you find yourself motivated to work out more because you want to look a certain way, I'm just glad you're moving more. You'll be healthier in the long run, and for me that's what matters.

As I said, different people respond to different methods.

But if you struggle with how you look, or you feel like society and social media promote nothing but a certain body and beauty type, and that affects your self-esteem to the point where you become unmotivated to exercise, I'd like you to think about something.

It's okay to feel down about how you look and use that as motivation to push harder.

It's also okay to love yourself exactly the way you are.

But I think *you can have it both ways.* You can love yourself as you are today and also push yourself toward better health tomorrow and the next day.

In a perfect world no one would worry about how they look. No one would worry about what other people think about how they look. But we don't live in that world.

No matter how you feel about your body and your self-worth, never let that get in the way of taking care of yourself.

I live and work within medical reality, and what I and my physician colleagues see every day is people not taking care of themselves and having serious, chronic health problems as a result.

So there's a conflict there. A person's desire to accept and love themselves as they are could result in health problems. The problems may not be there today. But they could be there tomorrow, and they will be there someday. It's virtually guaranteed.

That's why I encourage people to move more even if exercise in some forms makes them uncomfortable, or intimidates them, or makes them feel less-than because they don't look and perform a certain way.

Exercise truly does make everything better.

And when it comes to how you feel about yourself, you can love yourself today and push yourself to improve for tomorrow.

The Art of the Super-Simple Workout

Here's an experiment. I bet I can give you a total-body workout most Americans (and maybe even you) wouldn't be able to finish. And I can do it in less than fifty words.

After a ten-minute warm-up to light sweat . . .
 Do pushups for one minute. Rest one minute.
 Hold plank for one minute. Rest one minute.
 Do squats for one minute. Rest one minute.

Do mountain climbers for one minute. Rest one minute.
Repeat two more times.

That's a good thirty-minute workout that will kick the butts of most people. Six lines, forty-five words.

Of course, there are endless workout possibilities—sets and reps and progressions and daily logs, and never ever skip leg day. Fitness magazines used to publish foldout posters to detail one four-week strength-training plan *just for shoulders*.

Simple is simpler.

Have a look at this 2021 study from the *International Journal of Exercise Science:* Researchers had a group of inactive adults perform an eleven-minute workout three times a week for six weeks.[1] And talk about simple: Do a one-minute warm-up, then perform an exercise at a "challenging" pace for sixty seconds, rest for sixty seconds, then on to the next exercise. They did burpees, high knees, split squat jumps, high knees, squat jumps—and done. They moved at about 82 percent of their max heart rate and a perceived exertion of 14 out of 20. Compared with a control group that did nothing, these formerly inactive adults had significantly higher rates of VO2 output (oxygen use) and power output.

Two keys to that study: minimal time commitment and no equipment.

Just moving with purpose.

That's what we're talking about here. Simple is so effective.

When you're reawakening your body and falling back into love with movement, complex exercises and workouts just aren't necessary. The majority of people are not training to become elite athletes.

Movement is simple. If you're looking to fall back in love with movement, it's better to focus on something you really like—and could love.

The truth: You can change your body for the better by doing a handful of really good exercises.

You don't need to buy weights—unless you want to.

You don't need to join a gym—unless you want to.

You don't need to do elaborate workouts—unless you want to.

You don't need to spend a bunch of money—unless you want to. Keep it simple.

EXERCISE AS MEDICINE: WHAT'S THE MINIMUM REQUIRED DOSE?

It's smaller than you think. We've touched on this before, but a 2022 study in the *British Journal of Sports Medicine* looked at a national cohort survey of 416,000 U.S. adults.[2] The minimum dose: one hour per week of moderate to vigorous exercise for "significant mortality risk reduction." The benefits increased with more exercise, leveling off at three hours per week.

Why Boring Is Beautiful

You hear me say movement is simple. Here's the problem with simple. People hear "simple" and think "boring."

I could respond by saying a workout is only as boring as you make it. But there's something even more important to say: *With fitness, boring brings transformation.*

Here's yet another instance where behavioral economics—how your brain reacts to money—also applies to exercise and health. If you have a 401(k), I'm going to assume you know what a stock index fund is. The man who invented index investing is the late Jack Bogle, founder of Vanguard, the massive nonprofit mutual fund company. Bogle's investing philosophy was this: The average everyday person doesn't have time to research individual stocks, so he created a fund where each investor was exposed to the entire stock market. Steady deposits into your index fund over many years combining with the market's average annual return was the best way for ordinary people to grow serious wealth over time.

Contrast that with individual stock picking, holding stocks for a short gain then dumping them, buying a new, shiny thing, then playing around with more complicated methods like short selling, options, and the frenzy you see each day on investment channels—all of it tantamount to casino gambling. Some people do it. They love the adrenaline of it, and some remain convinced that they can "beat the market" and score more gains than active mutual fund managers.

Two mindsets: Bogle's simple, boring approach versus the gambler's adrenalized, shiny-new-thing approach.

Some fitness enthusiasts have the same mindset. Always trying a crazy new movement, looking out for the cool new thing, jumping on the new "science" someone just brought to light. They love the hype of it all.

Bogle sums up this mentality perfectly: "When we all speak of 'the stock market,' it's meaningless. It goes up and it goes down, but in the long run it goes up. The stock market, therefore, is noise. A giant distraction from the business of investing."[3]

I love that quote because you can apply it to fitness and wellness hype. All the fired-up influencers you see doing wild new exercises on social media are noise. They come, they go. A giant distraction from the business of health.

More Bogle: "I look at indexing as being simple, and sad to say, boring. That's good! Be bored by the process but elated by the outcome."

Now sub in "consistent exercise" for "indexing." That's how this works.

Be bored by the process but elated by the outcome.

Don't confuse simple with ineffective.

Don't conflate consistent with boring.

SIMPLICITY + CONSISTENCY + TIME = TRANSFORMATION

Your Movement Mindset

What are you thinking when you move?

We don't have to be talking about a workout. You could be doing chores. Cutting the grass. Vacuuming. Sometimes we concentrate on the task at hand. Sometimes our minds wander. That can be enjoyable or stressful, depending on what you're focusing on.

The point: No matter what we're doing, we're thinking while we do it.

What are you thinking when it's time to exercise? The folks with healthy motivation feel excitement or some other positive emotion. Or, even facing a workout in a down mood, a begrudging awareness that movement will make them feel better in the end.

Then there are the people who think beforehand, *This is gonna suck.*

During: *This sucks, this sucks, this sucks.*

After: *That sucked.*

My advice: Use all that thinking to your advantage. In the time you'll spend moving, be it a walk or climbing Everest, you'll have an opportunity to think a zillion thoughts.

Key word there: *opportunity.*

Your workout is an opportunity to completely shift your mindset and embrace all the good things you're doing and, very soon, thinking.

One helpful and very enjoyable method is mindfulness, consciously focusing so you're aware of what you're feeling in each moment. This doesn't have to be a formal thing. In fact, it may be most useful if you start out by setting your mind to measure appreciation as you go.

Appreciate yourself: You're doing it.

Appreciate your body: It's doing it.

Appreciate the moment, this stretch of time, the day, the weather: This is amazing.

Go out and move your body and forget it's exercise. It's just you, moving. And your body loves you for it. Even if it's just a simple walk, your body is responding from your brain to your feet with positive reactions, physical, chemical, psychological, all of them saying the same thing: This is good.

If you're strength-training, feel your muscles engage on every rep. That's also smart because it helps you maintain proper form. Pretty amazing what your body can do, huh? This is what you were built for.

This time is also about *connection.*

If you're with yourself, connect with yourself.

If you're with someone, connect with them.

If you're listening to music, connect with it.

If you're out in a park or somewhere scenic, connect with your surroundings.

I sometimes even connect with the ground while I'm running. Each foot strike I feel the ground; I feel how my foot rolls heel to toe, just pure rhythm and focus.

Now, of course your mind can wander while you move. Steady-state walking and running can be incredibly meditative.

This is what I mean by a healthy mindset. Engage. Feel your body work, your muscles perform. That's the real *why*.

And when you're finished? Stay engaged. Have a water and catch your breath and feel your heart rate come down and just feel how good it feels to have done what you just did.

Mindset can change everything.

You can be the "*This sucks*" person. Or you can just let go and allow yourself to enjoy this.

CHAPTER 11

The Best Exercises No One
Can Put a Price Tag On

I'm now going to show you a group of simple exercises. We'll also look at the history of these exercises—and that's deliberate—because I want you to understand that humans have been doing them for centuries, and in some cases millennia. These exercises deserve to be appreciated for their simplicity and power.

But let's head off something at the pass before we even get into it.

There are no "beginner" exercises. There are only fitness levels. If you're just starting out or have low- to mid-level fitness, your body can handle a certain amount of exercise before you overexert yourself, your muscles fail, and you risk injury. If you haven't tried a certain exercise before, sure, you can be considered a beginner in that sense. But the exercise itself? People with higher fitness levels do that exercise too.

Again, there are no beginner exercises, only fitness levels.

I emphasize that because when you see my exercise list, you might be thinking, *There has to be more to it. These exercises are so basic. They're too simple. I know all this already. How will it help?*

Stop. That line of thinking is a brick wall. Take what you just said one sentence at a time.

These exercises are so basic. They are more than basic. They are *foundational.* They are the bedrock of every exercise program ever devised.

They're too simple. Yes, not just simple, but effective. The vast majority of people with low- or medium-level fitness will see fantastic results from the most basic workouts.

I know all this already. Yes. And we now know how effective knowledge is when you don't use it.

How will it help? These exercises, combined simply and without any preciousness or self-importance, won't just help. They'll build a transformative fitness foundation. They will change your body and health.

Walking

You bet I'm beginning with the most fundamental form of human physical activity. Too simple? Too basic? Too boring? Then you aren't walking anywhere interesting.

Right now, researchers estimate that the first "person" to walk upright was *Ardipithecus ramidus,* or "Ardi." And those first steps happened about 4.4 million years ago.[1] *Homo erectus,* the more famous ancestor who grew taller with longer legs, arrived only about 1.9 million years ago. That's a long walk through the entirety of human history. Now it's your turn, and as Robin Williams says when reciting Walt Whitman in *Dead Poets Society,* "The powerful play goes on, and you may contribute a verse." The steps you take today mimic the steps all humans have taken for millions of years. A friend of mine recently took his son to Washington, D.C., for a weekend, and according to step count, they walked nineteen miles in two days just exploring the Mall and surrounding monuments and museums—the same steps millions of others have taken all the way back to the beginning of American history. Nearly eighty thousand steps between them and not a boring one among them.

Walking is our most basic form of exercise and ridiculously effective for improving health. Imagine taking the "ten thousand steps a day" advice to heart and doing so for an entire year. That's 3.65 million steps. And those steps will be uniquely *your* steps. Where will they take you?

As for the ol' ten thousand steps rule, it doesn't even have to be your rule. That number originated in Japan in 1965 when a company named Yamasa Clock manufactured a pedometer they called Manpo-kei, which translates to "ten thousand steps meter." Plus, 10K is a nice round number.

STAIRS ARE HIGH-QUALITY STEPS

A 2023 study in *Atherosclerosis* of more than 450,000 people found that those who climbed at least five flights of stairs (about fifty steps) daily had a 20 percent lower risk of atherosclerotic cardiovascular disease (which includes coronary artery disease and ischemic stroke).[2]

What number of steps has been medically recommended? Research varies, but it's much lower. A 2023 review of twelve studies covering 111,000 people in the *Journal of the American College of Cardiology* found "significant risk reductions" for cardiovascular disease starting at 2,700 steps and all-cause mortality at 2,500, with "optimum doses" being 8,800 and 7,100, respectively.[3] A 2022 meta-analysis of walking studies in *Lancet Public Health* encompassed more than forty-seven thousand people and found a gradually decreasing risk of mortality according to step count and age. Folks older than sixty enjoyed a steadily decreasing risk of death the more steps they took up until six thousand to eight thousand per day. Folks younger than sixty got similar benefits up through eight thousand to ten thousand steps per day.[4] So while 10K a day is a worthy goal, you still get health benefits with a lot fewer.

Whenever you need to move, the best advice echoes back 4.4 million years: *Take a walk.*

16,060,000,000,000

Number of steps one human ancestor would take if they got their ten thousand steps each day for 4.4 million years.

Running

Running is as old as walking. Those who ran survived. Eventually, running became recreational. Racing, for example, makes all the sense in the world because even the most primitive human can see if he or she is faster or slower than other humans. Those who ran *fastest* survived even longer, especially when you consider their longer lives gave them better mating potential for a longer time, producing off-spring who could run fast too. Running history certainly took a turn around 490 B.C. when a Greek soldier, Pheidippides, ran about twenty-five miles from Marathon to Athens with news of a military victory—and then died from the effort (no word if he broke 3:30). That tale, of course, is where marathons come from, which to this day are considered the elite distance running competitions. The Olympics added the marathon in 1896, and one year later the first marathon was run in Boston. Today, upwards of 1.3 million people run a 26.2-mile race each year worldwide. The stats on shorter dis-tances are probably more meaningful: About 9 million run 5K (3.1 miles) races in the United States each year too. There is no barrier to entry. Anyone can try it.

Running is my favorite thing. It's good for your lungs and heart. It's good for your bones. It's good for your brain *and* your mind. And contrary to what some people think, it's really good for your knees. I've blown out both my ACLs playing sports, and I've still run thou-sands of miles on those knees since then.

After millions of years, we're still running to live longer. If you can run, run. It's just about the perfect physical activity.

Doubled

Incidence of knee osteoarthritis in people age fifty and older since the mid-twentieth century indicates that our modern, sedentary lifestyle may contribute to our bones wearing down. When we were more ac-tive as a society—particularly preindustrial hunter-gatherers and farmers—our knees were healthier for longer into middle age.[5]

Pushup

The simplicity of the pushup is its perfection. Humans have been doing them for thousands of years, possibly as early as the Roman Empire and in training Hindu fighters in India. In fact, the military has adored the pushup as a basic training tool and disciplinary measure for decades, if not centuries (just ask Bill Murray in *Stripes*). Why? To do them, you need nothing more than a floor.

The initial thought most have is that the pushup is a chest exercise. Yes, it hits your pectorals, but so many more muscles and joints engage. Fingers and hands support your wrists, supporting your forearms, engaging your elbows and upper arms—triceps in particular—into your shoulders front and back. And then you're rigid from your neck to your toes. Think of the exercise as a plank with extreme upper-body benefits.

Pushups are hard. That's their genius. Simple and effective. Even if you can do a bunch, they will always wear you out. Take them as a tool, a challenge, a dare.

Or take them as a litmus test for cardiovascular disease risk. A *JAMA* study of more than 1,100 men with a ten-year follow-up found that those who could perform forty pushups or more had a 95 percent lower risk of a cardiovascular disease "event" than those who could do ten or fewer.[6] Short answer: The more pushups a person can do, the healthier that person tends to be.

And while we're on the subject of Bill Murray, in *Stripes* his pushup form is excellent—body rigid from head to toe, a full rep down to the ground and back up in a nonrushed manner. Too many folks out there are doing halfsie-reps real fast with haphazard form to boost their total. Quality is more important than quantity, folks. Drop and give yourself twenty (and work up to forty-plus).

Plank

Plank is the silent, immovable partner to the pushup—a core staple for your core. If you can't appreciate how effective they are, hold one for a minute. Then do twenty pushups. Your core will be burning more than your arms.

The key to the plank is engagement. Hold your body straight while pushing into the floor. Engage your core, sure, but every muscle head to toe. It's a fascinating experiment because it's the exact opposite of what we've been talking about in the book: movement. You don't move a centimeter, but every muscle screams.

Squat

The largest muscles you have reside in the lower body and are the key to maintaining mobility and athleticism as you age. People generally have the most problems in their lower body—like knee arthritis or plantar pain or hip issues—because they haven't kept their legs fit. The more you build your legs, the better you'll be able to perform in all areas.

Squats are the cornerstone for that. Again, classic and simple: Stand with your feet shoulder-width apart. Put your arms out in front of you, or over your head, or put your hands behind your head—all are fine—and lower your butt until your thighs are perpendicular to the ground. Hold for a beat, then rise. In that movement, you've hit every muscle in your lower body. You're also training your body to do something it has to do fairly often in everyday life.

Here's a fun challenge that almost always amazes those who try it: If you're just getting back to physical activity, do several sets of body-weight squats every other day for two weeks. Then grab a full laundry basket or grocery bags and walk up a flight of stairs. You will not believe the difference.

Eight hours or more

Time spent sitting each day will significantly raise your death and heart disease risk. In a 2022 *JAMA Cardiology* study of 105,000 people, those who sat for eight or more hours daily had a 17 to 50 percent higher risk of all-cause death and cardiovascular disease compared with those who sat for only four hours a day.[7]

Lunge

I love lunges and squats equally and think both are foundational. Lunges bring a bit more balance and coordination into the picture. This is another action that mimics everyday movement, but a fun bit of trivia is that the lunge is also one of the basic elements of fencing. You may not have everyday sword fights, but dedicated fencers are incredibly fit. This also goes to the history of the exercise—yet another one that goes back centuries.

The lunge is also incredibly variable. Forward, reverse, side to side, and you can even do "compass" lunges in continuous movement, hitting all points on the compass, including the diagonal ones. You can do walking lunges in all directions too, or you can stay in one place and alternate lunges with a jump.

You'll build powerful legs that way, but I like to think that the dynamic flexibility you develop in your lower body and the balance required are the real benefits of lunges. They are one of the best lower-body mobility exercises ever invented.

IS STANDING GOOD EXERCISE?

It's sneaky good. Standing is always better than sitting, for starters. But if you want a surprise, try this: The next time you have a phone or Zoom call when you would normally sit and talk, stand for the duration of the call instead—but put yourself on speaker and hold something heavy in front of you the entire time (a medicine ball is ideal, but even a big book or backpack full of books will work). One rule: Remain standing and don't put the object down. After ten to fifteen minutes you will know how good just standing and holding something can be.

Walking—but Better

As good as walking can be, adding weight to any walk makes it better. There are several ways you can do that.

Carries are as old as humans working with tools—particularly buckets to transport water. The Farmer's Carry is just that: picking up a heavy object in each hand and walking while carrying the objects at your sides (see Part Four for a more detailed description). In a gym, that could be a big dumbbell. At home, that could be jugs or buckets of water. All you need is something heavy and some space to walk. Try twenty paces forward and backward to your starting point and see how it feels. Hits every muscle, I promise you.

Other carries: overhead, in front of your chest, one-armed variations. Just get that heavy object from point A to point B.

Then there's another human evolutionary staple: rucking. Again, so simple. All you do is walk with a backpack full of weight, imitating early humans who figured out how to carry food and firewood and children on their backs. If that's not a good enough pedigree, understand that rucking is the foundational training strategy of the military—hiking with a full kit. You can buy weighted plates especially made for rucking, or just stuff your backpack full of books. The point is to add more effort to something you're already doing. Try it next time you walk your dog.

Ten seconds

Time spent standing on one leg to lower your risk of death. A 2021 *British Journal of Sports Medicine* study of 1,700 older adults for twelve years found that nearly 18 percent of those who could not balance on one leg for ten seconds died during the study, compared with 5 percent of those who could.[8] One-legged balance tests are an effective test for physical fitness in older people.

And of Course, There's More

Workouts, workouts, everywhere workouts. Swimming, cycling, rowing, yoga, martial arts, dance, hiking, team sports, solo sports, balls and sticks and gloves and pads and pucks. And gear: dumbbells, kettlebells, jump rope, core sliders, medicine balls, suspension trainers, and more and more and more. And gyms: box gyms and boutique gyms and sprawling sports performance facilities complete with sprint tracks and climbing walls.

It's all there—if you want it.

But when it comes to doing what we're doing right here—remembering what it was like to be in love with movement—it's nice to just get back to basics.

If you want to build anything, you have to start with a strong foundation. Now you have one. And if you've been reading between the lines, you can feel how just appreciating these simple movements makes them even more attractive as activities. These wonderful exercises exist, and you get to do them anytime you want. I *love* that. If you ever find yourself pausing and wondering, *What should I do,* start with a nice brisk walk interspersed with some lunges or pushups—and build from there.

CHAPTER 12

How the Plan Works

Way back in chapter 1, I said that it would be super-easy for me to tell you to "push yourself" and live healthier. Why not? Nike's been telling us to "just do it" for decades now. But we know that won't work. Proper motivation is deeply individual, as you've learned, and some people need more resources than others.

Remember also that I want you to push your mind *and* your body.

That's what this section is all about. This is the four-week plan that can formalize your approach to pushing yourself through hard moments. It will help you learn to become comfortable pushing yourself.

We've focused on physical activity in this book because that's my thing, and you'll see that focus continue in the following chapters. But you'll also quickly see that this plan can be applied to any situation.

It's simple: The plan is designed to make you consistently push for positive movement. That's all. No "lose 20 pounds in 4 weeks" or "one month to a sexy butt." Just consistency. I want you to become comfortable pushing yourself. I want pushing yourself to become routine.

Here's where we go from theory to practice.

"How Do I Push Myself?"

Fair question, the one we've been building up to. Literally, in the moment, how do I push myself? *What do I do?*

The most common answer might come from athletics—do one more lap, one more rep, find that next gear, that next level—you know that rap. That can work for some, but not everyone responds to the athletic coaching mindset. Not everyone has a coach watching what they do and encouraging them (even in their minds).

Pushing isn't routine or comfortable for you yet. So you need an easy way to pause the negative motivation and push through to the positive. It's a two-step process—and even though the explanation here takes time to read, these steps will happen in seconds in your mind.

Step 1: Pause.
Step 2: Prompt.

In moments of doubt, pause and ask yourself a simple question: *Why am I giving in?*

Something is lacking, either knowledge, belief, or emotion. Or a combination. Let's be real, though. Knowledge is usually the least of the problems. You know what to do in most situations. Usually some emotional response shakes your belief. *Yes, I know I had a workout scheduled in fifteen minutes, but I'm really busy and tired, and skipping one day won't matter.*

Boom, just like that, your perception of the situation has changed. "Skipping one day won't matter." You're perceiving it to be just fine to blow off your workout. That shift in perception gives you an emotional break because it relieves guilt.

Asking, "Why am I giving in?" allows for a quick analysis—and yes, this kind of analysis takes seconds because in most cases you know *exactly* why you're leaning toward the unhealthy choice. Doing the unhealthy thing will give you relief in some way, or pleasure, or escape.

Why am I giving in?

The more you pause to understand what's driving you the wrong way, the easier it'll be to course-correct. Also, I'll bet cash money that you'll begin to see repeating patterns (certain times of day, certain excuses, certain people, certain urges) that become easier to predict.

The result? The more you ask yourself, "Why am I giving in?," the more you'll learn to answer, "I'm not."

And you won't.

The immediate second step is the prompt. That's something you use to push yourself through the negative motivation. Some of your best prompts will sprout from all the information we've been talking about so far.

The Perfect Prompt

Behavioral activation might be the best of all: Get moving. The less you think about it, the better.

Still, we humans like to complicate simple things, so it's possible that you need some kind of trigger to set your behavioral activation in motion. It can be creative or silly or unique, as long as it *works*.

The key: Your behavioral activation prompt needs to be immediate. A mantra. A ritual. A routine. Maybe it's just recognizing it's time, it's necessary, it's the thing to do right now. Maybe it's firing up a certain piece of music or a certain movie clip. Maybe it's whispering to yourself, "This is something good just for me," or maybe "No one ever regretted a good workout," and hey, even "Just do it" is fine if it gets you moving. Remember my friend Jane's "I get to do this."

Or it could be a simple physical act, like turning your back on the refrigerator before you open it. I know a woman who makes a ritual of tying her shoes before working out. It sets her mind.

When you think of the three motivational ingredients—knowledge, emotion, belief—you can't sit around and hope that on any given day they line up in perfect harmony and the sun shines on you and you head out the door for a workout. Maybe some days they will. But you know most days they won't.

Behavioral activation is an effective way to force your emotions and belief into line. If they're in a negative or neutral state, pushing yourself to start a workout will then push those emotions and belief into positive ranges.

Behavioral activation is you in full control. You own the narrative ("I'm gonna work out today and feel great"), you choose the time and place, you reject the negative motivations. Every positive thing you feel as a result of that workout—that's *you*. You did that.

That's pushing yourself.

That's doing the right thing—not because you feel up to it, but because you don't.

Recalculate Your Cost to Act

Now's the time to use all those cost-to-act accounting tricks to keep you focused.

Add anticipation. Have something fun waiting for you during today's workout. Favorite band has a new album. Favorite podcast has a new episode. Favorite author has a new audiobook. Meet a friend or spouse or date or other person you can't wait to see for the session.

Incentivize. Place a bet with friends or even yourself. Finally, get some skin in your game.

Gamify. Make it a competition. No one around? Compete with yourself and try to beat your previous workout's results.

Control. Think of all the reasons a workout will help you distance yourself from a scary health outcome. That's you taking the wheel and driving your own well-being, how fit you are, how successfully you age, how good you feel going forward. You get to control that, and it's an amazing accomplishment.

Keep going. Invent your own. You can devise dozens of ways to make your cost to act "worth it."

Use the Big List

This list is a simple way to organize what we worked through along the way here, to assemble the blind spots and pain points in one place.

If you're striving to push yourself to make good choices and are, say, hitting a wall or feeling your resolve flag, all you need to do is think back to the Big List and which items mess with you the most.

You can also use it for deeper thought when you have more time to work through real problem areas. Combine the Big List with the self-test from chapter 3, and you have a pretty sharp set of tools to pinpoint where and how you're struggling. You'll be able to spot what you're dealing with, or what you can take away, or how to re-boot. Plus, that will be coupled with all the good things you already have in place, like the knowledge of how good movement is for you, the progress you've already made, and what's possible in the future. Those are not small things.

We don't need to rehash each item on the list since we spoke about almost all of them in detail previously in the book. But here I'm adding some simple questions you can ask yourself if you find yourself struggling with one or more of them.

As I've said before, all you need to do is be honest with your answers.

The Big List

1. **Biases.** What cognitive biases do I recognize in myself? How do they hold me back? Am I willing to change my behavior when I see their negative effects? If not, why not? Why do I have such a hard time admitting something isn't working?
2. **Perception.** Do I tend toward negative or positive perception of healthy choices? How do I perceive myself? Can I honestly say my self-perceptions are objectively accurate? Am I really the person I think I am—or is there something better?
3. **Incentives.** What rewards make me want to make healthy choices? Rewards for minute-to-minute behavior aside, what other long-term benefits could I enjoy if I push for a healthier lifestyle?
4. **Knowledge.** If I know what I need to do to make healthy choices, why don't I do it?

5. **Curiosity.** What shuts down my natural curiosity, and what wakes it up? Am I willing to learn something new, even if it challenges what I currently believe? How could encouraging a hunger for healthier knowledge and behavior change my life?

6. **Self-esteem.** Do I feel I'm objective when I judge myself? Am I too harsh? What choices can I make that will make me feel better about myself? Am I prepared to feel better about myself?

7. **Self-efficacy.** Do I underestimate myself? What do I believe I am capable of?

8. **Control.** How do I feel when I have control over my lifestyle versus little or no control? What changes can I make that will give me more control?

9. **Community.** Who can I count on to push me forward and upward, and how can I find more of those people? Am I willing to reach out and connect with new people? Am I willing to move away from those who hold me back?

10. **(It's a secret—keep reading.)**

The truth is, each item on the list could inspire a hundred questions. My suggestion to you: When you think about new healthy choices and feel a natural resistance in your mind, for any reason, allow the healthy voice inside to speak up. And listen to it.

That's where the questions that apply most to you will come from.

That's where the most personal answers will come from too.

Starting the Four-Week Plan

Think about your garden-variety four-week diet/eating plan or four-week fitness plan. Each day the plan says, "Here's what to eat when" or "Here's your workout for the day down to sets, reps, and rest." What makes them so useful? They tell you exactly what to do.

Aside from the actual work involved in execution, they're remarkably simple. That's my goal with the Push plan as well.

In fact, you may look at the four-week grid and think, *Is that all?*

Don't be deceived by the simplicity of the plan. The simplicity is the point, the same way keeping workouts simple is the point. This plan asks: Can you stick to it and increase your positive behavior over time? Can you reach a point where you feel comfortable pushing yourself past unhealthy motivation in any moment?

If you look at this plan and think it's too simple, well, see if you can complete it. That's not a dare, and neither is the plan. It is a test, however, and it's help.

Four weeks is not a magical time frame. It's a manageable one.

The plan links to what I said about how I tell my patients to set goals. It has to be challenging, a little bigger than what you're comfortable with, and even a little scary.

I used two processes that I'm intimately familiar with to create the plan framework. The first is injury rehabilitation. Think about how an injured patient rehabs. A steady build, increasing activity and intensity—pushing yourself past a comfort zone, of course—from physical therapy to gradual return to full activity. You're able to do more and more as you improve. So, if it helps, think of this four-week plan as your "rehab" plan, but you're rehabilitating your mindset.

I also designed the plan with marathon training in mind. This is not a sprint. Four weeks isn't short, but it's not long either. Like marathon training, there's a steady build here. Some days will be more focused than others, by design. But you will face increasing "positive" activity as you go. The goal is to set up a structure for success, a way for you to learn how to push yourself—but also to keep the idea of pushing yourself top-of-mind even in the moments when the plan doesn't ask you to.

How it works: On certain days you need to push through negative motivation to achieve positive motivation and execute a healthy choice.

What counts as a "push"? The point of the book is not just to make positive choices. I want you to learn to master your fitness motivation. You need to learn to push through the negative impulses too. So for a "push" to count for the day, it needs to be consequential and it needs to reverse negative motivation. I don't view, say, swapping a Pop-Tart for a Greek yogurt first thing in the morning as a consequential push if it means you skip a workout later because you count dodging a Pop-Tart as your push for the day. The skipped workout is far more consequential. If you find yourself playing games like this with the plan, you're not taking it to heart and you remain in a negativity loop.

How do you keep track? For physical activity, your phone does that for you already: step count, stairs climbed, workout duration, and so on. If you have a smartwatch synched to your phone, you can record just about any type of workout. Use the tech you have.

For the other choices you have to make within a day, what you track and how closely you need to is up to you. Free food and habit trackers exist, and at this point in humanity's timeline, technology is probably the way to go. But hey, if you want to go old-school and use a spreadsheet or little notebook or food diary, I encourage the throwback. It all works.

The plan is illustrated in a basic grid—with tons of extra information you can use to make things even better. The grid tells you how many positive actions you need to push yourself to take that day. Some days require more than others. The frequency increases as the weeks go by. Again, this is all about becoming comfortable pushing yourself.

Here's how this plan grid works:

On "0" days: Do your thing. Give yourself a break.

On "+1" days: Push in one serious way against negative tendencies to achieve positive movement. For example, let's say you have a workout planned and something intervenes, making it easy for you to say, "I'll skip it today." On a +1 day, you would push back against this negative tendency and do the workout, or even an abbreviated workout. That's your +1 for the day—you pushed yourself and did the right thing.

On "+2" days: Push in at least two serious ways against negative tendencies to achieve positive movement. Example: The workout dilemma we just talked about plus a second scenario where a third (or fourth) glass of weeknight wine and a late hour are calling your name. On a +2 day, you push back against two negative tendencies and do the healthy thing.

On "+3" days: Push in at least three serious ways. These days should be very close to full-on Push days. The best advice here is to keep things simple: Your brain pushes you to an unhealthy craving, you consciously push back. How do you know what makes a "negative tendency"? Your knowledge—you know what's good for you and what isn't because you've been living that way a long time and now want to change. I focus on fitness motivation, but unhealthy motivation can cut across a lot of activities. If you find yourself erring toward old tendencies, pause and prompt. Do the healthy thing.

On Push days: You are mindful all day of negative motivations and push back against them, pushing ahead with positive responses and behavior. It's *your* day, you do not let up.

WEEK	MON	TUE	WED	THU	FRI	SAT	SUN
1	0	PUSH	+1	+2	0	+1	PUSH
2	0	PUSH	+2	+2	+1	+1	PUSH
3	+1	PUSH	+2	+3	+1	+2	PUSH
4	PUSH	PUSH	+1	PUSH	+1	PUSH	PUSH
5+			EVERY DAY IS A PUSH DAY				

The simplicity is the magic trick here: You will do it, or you won't.

You already know what happens if you don't. You're living it right now.

This is about consistency: doing it when you need to and gradually reaching a point of frequency and routine where you do it because it clicks with you, it makes sense, it feels normal. I stop short of using the word *habit,* as a habit suggests you no longer need to think about doing it, and with healthy choices it's safer to lean toward an active rather than passive approach.

That's it. You don't have to count calories or sets and reps or running mileage (unless that's your thing). You just have to push when needed. You have to show up. And here's a neat thing: You'll find that your heavier push days will produce a halo effect across your lighter days where you'll start to push when you need to even though the plan doesn't require it (some call it spillover effect). Once that starts to happen, you're golden. That means you're becoming more conscious of how and when you need to push. You're more comfortable pushing yourself.

That's where you want to be.

CHAPTER 13

Weeks 1 Through 4

WEEK 1

MON	TUE	WED	THU	FRI	SAT	SUN
0	PUSH	+1	+2	0	+1	PUSH

Week 1 features only two full-on Push days. Wednesday, Thursday, and Saturday you'll have to pick the particular occasions where you want to push yourself. The easiest thing to do is plan those occasions around physical activity. A healthy, consequential push doesn't have to be centered on exercise, but the focus of this book has been movement, so it makes the most sense—after all, you don't just want to get comfortable pushing yourself, you want to fall back in love with movement. Just be careful to avoid the aforementioned Pop-Tart trap of blowing off your workout later because "I already used my Push moment for the day."

And right there is one of the secrets of this plan I hope you embrace: These moments and days when the plan tells you to push through are the bare minimums. Push yourself to push yourself. If you can, do more than you need to.

The more you do it, the more comfortable you'll be doing it, and the more automatic it will all become.

Some Helpful Tips for the First Week

If you're strength-training, focus on the movement. Focus on how your body moves and muscles engage. This serves two purposes: For formal exercises you need to focus on the quality of your form, especially if you're just getting back into working out. A good rule to go by is that *the quality of your reps is more important than the quantity.* This prevents injury. The second purpose is keeping your mind engaged in what you're doing. There's nothing wrong with a wandering mind while walking or running—steady-state exercise can be meditative that way—but an appreciation of your body and what it can do can be really satisfying and make you want to come back to exercise even more.

Prepare for increased appetite. This is not a weight loss book. This is a book about healthy motivation and movement. But know this: If you increase your physical activity, your body may crave more calories as fuel. Because of this, you could find that you feel stronger and fitter from exercise, but the numbers on the scale don't move favorably. One way to understand it: Even if you burn five hundred calories from a really good workout and you say, "I earned this" when eyeing a plate of food, you can consume *more* than five hundred calories in just a few minutes, maybe even a few bites. Generally speaking, exercise is not an ideal weight loss tool (though you can lose weight by increasing your activity). Exercise is far more effective for better health, vitality, and longevity. If you're looking to lose weight, you'll have to watch what you eat as well. I wish there were shortcuts here, but if there were, we'd all use them.

A Sample Fifty-Word Workout

Each week I'll offer you a sample workout—but I'll reiterate that you don't have to do anything other than walking or other activities that make you happy. That said, resistance exercises have incredible benefits, so consider them.

And these fifty-word workouts are ideal for Push days or when you want to change things up, challenge yourself, or get a new activity fast (you can put together your own fifty-word workout in about thirty seconds if you use Part Four in the back of the book).

For week 1, this sample is loaded with the basics because I'd prefer you work on basic things rather than get stuck overthinking what you should do. Do the basics, enjoy the basics, embrace the basics—that's a good when-in-doubt rule. The basics are always there and will always work for you.

For more info on how to make this workout easier/harder or to see exercise descriptions, go to Part Four.

Warm-up five to ten minutes
  Pushups (page 173) for one minute / Rest for one minute
  Squats (page 180) for one minute / Rest for one minute
  Plank (page 188) for one minute / Rest for one minute
  Shuttle run (page 192) for one minute / Rest for one minute
  Repeat this circuit three times

Bonus Help: Let's Talk About Time

This is a good time to contemplate time.

The benefits of proper motivation are obvious, and we've gone over them. I personally don't believe we can undervalue healthspan. And keeping yourself pointed in the right direction brings a host of benefits, as we've seen. But there's one more benefit I wanted to save until now. It may be the biggest value on investment and perhaps the most unexpected: *time.*

This might seem counterintuitive since you must *take* time to add regular physical activity to your day, eat well, and interact with others. But in my experience, that relatively small time investment pays massive quality-of-life dividends by raising the value of every other hour of your day.

If time is money, here's how to "follow the money," so to speak:

- Getting fitter improves physical capability, making you more effective at even mundane chores. Home life improves.
- Healthier choices raise your mental performance, making you better at your job. Work life improves.
- Improved self-efficacy brings a healthier mindset, making you better at personal interaction, reacting to stress, and

maintaining positivity. Relationships across the board
improve.

- General wellness can result in weight loss and positive
  physical changes. How others perceive you will improve.
- All of these things boost energy levels. You'll get better at
  everything because you'll perform at a higher level for a
  longer period of time.

Now, I know all about the "I have no time to exercise" bit. You probably have your own version of it, because just about everyone does. I don't have time either, but I exercise anyway. Why? If I'm honest with myself, the time really is there if I look—and if it isn't, I can steal some.

That's why I'm fine with this item from the sorry-not-sorry file: If you say, "I don't have time to exercise," what you really don't have is credibility.

Everyone is busy.

Everyone has time for physical activity at some point in their day.

Both of those statements can be true.

Analyses of the American Time Use Survey are always revealing, and numbers don't lie. COVID-19 changed our lives in many ways, and time use is one of them. Now that so many of us work remotely or hybrid, the American Time Use Survey shows we've collectively freed up sixty million hours commuting each day.[1] What are we doing with that time? The number one answer is "leisure at home," and the runner-up is "sleeping."

Here's a kicker, though: Even before the pandemic, we were flush with extra time. A Centers for Disease Control and Prevention study published in 2019 looked at the American Time Use Survey and found the average American had more than five hours of leisure time a day and that no subgroup of people had less than four and a half.[2] Which means that even back then a thirty-minute workout took up exactly 10 percent of your leisure time. I'm sure many people would say, "Wow, I sure don't feel like I have five hours to spare each day," and maybe you don't, but this is an easy audit.

Just be honest. Even the busiest of us have time to move. That's why it's so critical to always think of the benefits.

The time you spend engaged in things like purposeful movement can be meditative and useful. You can focus on the moment. You can think on problems, goals, and plans. You can listen to audiobooks and podcasts. You can take yourself outside and exercise in nature. You can try bibliotherapy, art therapy, culinary therapy. The point is, the time you spend on healthy activities has measurable value and brings similar value to the rest of your day.

Remember, movement is cumulative. Exercise snacks count.

All of this adds up to a better quality of life across the board: relationships, career, money, definitions of success, and more.

Enjoy your first week!

WEEK 2

MON	TUE	WED	THU	FRI	SAT	SUN
0	PUSH	+2	+2	+1	+1	PUSH

In week 2 we go from two off days to just one. This is not a massive increase and will keep you on track, so pushing yourself claims just a little bit more real estate in your mind. As I mentioned, I designed these weeks to mimic marathon training, gradual increases over time, but as with marathon training, no matter how much effort you expend in a given week, the idea of the push never leaves your brain.

By now, the need to push yourself should be firmly entrenched and you've had a week to acclimate to doing it with semiregularity. Now you know how it feels. This week you'll do it a bit more.

Some Helpful Tips for Week 2

A quick word about alcohol. Four words, to be exact: You don't need it. Drinking can serve many purposes in our minds, some legitimate, some not. For example, there's nothing wrong with having a drink or two with friends. But speaking as a physician, I think there may be no subject that causes patients to lie to doctors more about how much they do a thing. And that's the false part: People are rarely honest with themselves and others about how much they drink. So consider how your drinking holds you back from this particular mission, falling in love with movement again.

Excessive drinking sabotages healthy motivation. No drunk person ever craved a salad. No hungover person ever said, "I can't wait to work out."

More on how healthier habits work all the way down to the cellular level. Epigenetics, the study of how lifestyle affects our genes, may ultimately be the field that determines future breakthroughs in human longevity. A study review in *Cell Metabolism* summarized the recent epigenetic data on obesity and type 2 diabetes and found that good habits bring positive "epigenetic variation" to fat tissue, skeletal muscle, pancreatic and liver function, and blood health.[3] Healthy habits = healthier genes.

A Sample Fifty-Word Workout

The exercises get a little more unique this week, but the ultimate total-body balance is still there. Hip raises may be one of the best glute exercises, and anyone who knows me knows one of my best pieces of advice is "A strong butt is the key to a happy life." A strong butt helps mitigate lower back pain and is a key part of your posterior kinetic chain, the muscles on the back half of your body from your shoulders down to your heels that interact and support each other in complex movements.

For more info on how to make this workout easier/harder or to see exercise descriptions, go to Part Four.

> *Warm-up five to ten minutes*
>> *Bench dip (page 177) for one minute / Rest for one minute*
>> *Single-leg deadlift reach (page 182) for one minute / Rest for one minute*
>> *Hip raise (page 189) for one minute / Rest for one minute*
>> *Inchworms (page 173) for one minute / Rest for one minute*
>> *Repeat this circuit three times*

Bonus Help: Let's Talk About Intensity

I'm a fan of exercise intensity. In many ways intensity is the essence of what it means to push your mind and body. You have to really work to achieve it. You have to *want* to get there. Isn't that what we've been talking about since page 1?

In short, the more intensity, the more benefits you get from the workout. You may have heard of HIIT workouts, or high-intensity interval training, where you work in short, full-on bursts of activity. When I discovered HIIT, it was a revelation.

I understand you may be just starting out or getting back into physical activity, and I most certainly have been saying that a daily walk is all you need for health benefits. All true! But a brisk walk instead of a slow walk works your heart and lungs harder. And you get where you're going faster—in every sense of the meaning.

Those are the two main "extra" benefits of intensity:

—**It's really good for you.** You put in more effort and your body works harder. This can increase the health benefits of whatever activity you do. Example: A 2022 *European Heart Journal* study looked at the physical activity of more than eighty-eight thousand people and found that higher intensity was associated with a 14 percent lower heart disease risk.[4] The folks who engaged in "moderate to vigorous" activity—the equivalent of doing a fourteen-minute walk in seven minutes—got the most benefit.

SHORTER INTENSE WORKOUTS = LONGER BRAIN BENEFITS

If you adopt HIIT-style workouts as a permanent part of your exercise plan and keep them going long term, the health benefits may extend as well, even if you eventually stop—particularly if you're older. A 2024 study in *Aging and Disease* put 151 older adults (ages sixty-five to eighty-five) through different long-term exercise programs and found that participants who did an HIIT program for six months saw a decrease in age-related brain shrinkage in "several cortical regions," in particular the hippocampus.[5] They also enjoyed increased connectivity between neural networks. No other exercise group experienced these results. HIIT increased or preserved cognitive ability, and here's the most surprising part: The effects were still measured five years later after the HIIT sessions stopped (not that I recommend stopping them once you start).

There's more: Hard-charging activity may benefit us on a cellular level. A small 2023 study in *Nutrients* found that high-intensity exercise raised the body's "scavenging" of reactive oxygen species (ROS) by 178 percent.[6] ROS cause oxidative damage in our cells—not a good thing—and the harder workouts increased the body's ability to eliminate ROS compared with lower-intensity exercise.

Intensity also helps increase mitochondrial volume (your cells' energy centers), deepens cardiovascular fitness, and strengthens muscles. It's a sweet cycle: The harder you work your body, the harder your body will be able to work.

—**Efficiency.** Working harder means you can compress the same amount of activity into a shorter time span with greater health benefits. For those who lament "not having time" to exercise, even a ten-minute session of hard intensity is beneficial.

Intensity can also help you improve your performance in less intense activities. For example, since forever, distance runners have used interval (sprint) training to increase their cardiovascular fitness and long-distance performance.

But honestly, when it comes down to the moment of working and sweating, you can just instinctively tell all these things about intensity. You feel it. And when you ramp up your intensity slowly so your body can adjust, and add more and more intensity over time to certain workouts, you just know. And you won't want to go back.

WEEK 3

MON	TUE	WED	THU	FRI	SAT	SUN
+1	PUSH	+2	+3	+1	+2	PUSH

Pushing yourself happens on some level every single day in week 3. This means you're thinking about it daily and becoming more comfortable with it. And even if it's not quite habit yet, you're feeling the positive effects. Your physical activity is still challenging, but maybe you've been able to increase your effort or volume. And you should also be noticing improvements, even if it's just a little easier to climb a flight of stairs.

Week 3 is also smack-dab in the "middle part" (remember that?). This is not a time to fall back. Keep going. You're learning every single day why we call it "pushing" yourself. You have to work at it. *Do the work.*

Some Helpful Tips for Week 3

A nice thought about aging. Longevity researchers have a unique term for health as we grow older: *successful aging*. That's a terrific goal. We've already talked about how physical activity and an active life in general give people an aging advantage over those who are sedentary. No matter how old you are right now, your future self will thank you for the sweat you work up today. Here's to aging successfully.

A new measure to monitor. You probably know your weight and maybe even your blood pressure and cholesterol, but you might want to pay attention to a number that could be as important as it is easy to measure: your waist-to-height ratio.

A study in *PLOS One* found this number to be more predictive of years lost than body mass index, as it focuses on more dangerous belly fat. Researchers recommend a waist circumference of less than half your height.[7] For example: If you're five feet eight inches tall (sixty-eight inches), measure your waist with the tape across your belly button. If it's less than thirty-four inches, you're good. If not, there's your goal.

A Sample Fifty-Word Workout

For more info on how to make this workout easier/harder or to see exercise descriptions, go to Part Four.

> *Warm-up five to ten minutes*
>> *Change-up pushups (page 175) for one minute /*
>>> *Rest for one minute*
>> *Reverse lunge with toe touch (page 184) for one minute /*
>>> *Rest for one minute*
>> *Bicycle crunch (page 190) for one minute /*
>>> *Rest for one minute*
>> *High knees (page 192) for one minute /*
>>> *Rest for one minute*
>> *Repeat this circuit three times*

Bonus Help: Let's Talk About Injuries

I've been a sports medicine physician for more than twenty years, and the one thing I can say is, *If you get hurt . . . KEEP MOVING.*

Now, I don't mean that if you pull a hamstring you should keep running or that if you think you've sprained your ankle playing pickleball you should finish out the game. (I'm fanatical about exercise, but not crazy!)

What I do mean: An injury is not a vacation from physical activity. In fact, as a doctor, I believe that suggesting "total rest" after an injury isn't just bad advice but bad medicine. You can certainly rest the body part that needs to heal, but keep moving. There are smart ways you can exercise without aggravating your injury, but you have to remain committed to staying active even though the ouch has taken some wind out of your sails. Don't think of it as "playing through the pain." Think of it as playing *around* the pain.

WHAT'S THE DIFFERENCE BETWEEN NORMAL EXERCISE PAIN AND INJURY?

World War II and Korean War hero General Lewis Puller is reportedly the genius behind the following quote you may have heard if you played high school sports: "Pain is weakness leaving the body." Inspirational, perhaps, but not really true. How should you approach pain when working out?

Exercise can cause discomfort while you're doing it and soreness after the fact, sometimes for as much as a day or two. This is especially true for people starting out. You should expect that. But does pain mean you're injured? No. Normal discomfort and pain subside. Injury pain doesn't, however, at least not right away. If you pull a muscle, you'll know it as soon as it grabs and the pain will force you to stop. A good rule of thumb: If pain persists in one area or if you experience any kind of joint weakness or instability, see a doctor. If you feel a pop or a tear, experience swelling or bruising, or joint range of motion is compromised, see a doctor. If persistent pain doesn't respond to at-home treatments like ice and rest, see a doctor.

Exercise doesn't just make you feel good. It keeps you from feeling bad. Even if your activity is limited, that's better than nothing. You won't lose all of your fitness progress. You'll get your health benefits. You'll feel better, be more positive, and keep smiling in spite of that little ding. An injury isn't the end of the world, or even the end of anything, if you approach fitness with patience and smarts.

Use what I call "dynamic rest."

First, rest and rehab your injury. Lay off that body part and do what's required to get it back to full strength. That could mean home-based remedies or seeing a doctor and using other prescribed interventions. Take your injury seriously.

Second? Dynamic means *in motion,* so *keep moving* while the rest and rehab go on. Use the following strategies:

- **Do something that doesn't aggravate the injury.** If you sprain your ankle, focus on upper-body and core work for a couple of weeks. If you hurt your shoulder, hit your lower body and core. Any upper-body injury means more walking and running in your future.
- **Go hard.** Whatever your "limited" activity may be, push yourself. You want your heart pounding and lungs heaving. You want to proceed as if the next level is inevitable. Because here's a crazy notion: You could even improve

your cardiovascular health—as well as whichever body zone you're working—during your injury rehab. Imagine being fitter after you heal.

And if you want to prevent injury? Or keep yourself from being hurt again?

- **Avoid the "terrible too's."** That would be doing too much, too hard, too soon. That goes for anything but is especially true for you walkers and runners. Pro sports teams employ "load monitoring" to make sure an athlete isn't overtraining. You should do the same. In a 2022 study published in the *British Journal of Sports Medicine,* my colleagues and I evaluated injury risk in 735 runners training for the New York City Marathon.[8] We found that, of all the modifiable factors like body weight or number of marathons completed, the strongest predictor of injury was rapidly increasing training miles. This was true for all levels, from novices to experienced runners. I suggest walkers and runners of all ability levels focus on slow, steady progression. While some runners can handle a more rapid mileage buildup, a 5 percent mileage increase per week is safer for most.

Everyone stumbles, twists, jerks, falls, and overexerts themselves. The key is to understand how injury works and listen to your body. But as I said, an injury is not a vacation from physical activity.

WEEK 4

MON	TUE	WED	THU	FRI	SAT	SUN
PUSH	PUSH	+1	PUSH	+1	PUSH	PUSH

WEEK 5+	EVERY DAY IS A PUSH DAY

This is the fourth and final week, but also the last week before the first week—that fifth week that turns you loose upon the world with better motivational skills. You'll be pushing just about every day now and will indeed push every day after week 4 ends.

Here's how to think about week 5 and beyond.

You know what it takes to push yourself effectively. You know when you have to. That's new knowledge.

You know how it makes you feel. New positive emotions.

You know what you're now capable of. New belief.

See how it all ties together in the end?

But it's not the end. You're just getting started. Aren't you curious to see what you can accomplish long term? I am. Let all the items of the Big List guide you forward—your curiosity, your self-efficacy, and more. Your life is out there, and all you need to navigate it is right here.

Some Helpful Tips for Week 4

An underrated health benefit of exercise. Your liver needs your help—and physical activity is the answer. A lesser-known but deadly serious "silent" health problem is nonalcoholic fatty liver disease (NAFLD)—recently renamed metabolic dysfunction–associated steatotic liver disease (MASLD). Up to 35 percent of U.S. adults have it right now, and it can eventually lead to liver failure.[9] Being sedentary, no matter how much you weigh, makes NAFLD worse over time. And yet research shows it responds extremely well to exercise in several ways: preventing fat from forming, oxidizing fat that is there, and reducing liver cell damage from the condition.[10] Even if we don't need another reason to exercise regularly, there always seems to be one.

What's your "Columbo move"? Next time you exercise, add a

Columbo move. What's that? If you've ever watched *Columbo*, you know he always has "just one more thing" for any murder suspect he questions. And it's always a zinger meant to expose the criminal. For your workout, when you're finishing up, just add "one more thing" to give that session a final extra boost. Maybe it's a brief sprint at the end of a run or a quick set of mountain climbers, anything that gives your workout a little Columbo action at the end. Remember: All exercise is cumulative and adds up in the long run.

A Sample Fifty-Word Workout

For more info on how to make this workout easier/harder or to see exercise descriptions, go to Part Four.

> *Warm-up five to ten minutes*
> > *Floor Y-T-I raises (page 176) for one minute / Rest for one minute*
> > *Squat jump (page 182) for one minute / Rest for one minute*
> > *Elevated bird dog (page 189) for one minute / Rest for one minute*
> > *Burpee with pushup (page 193) for one minute / Rest for one minute*
> > *Repeat this circuit three times*

Bonus Help: Let's Talk About Recovery

When you start exercising regularly, recovery is critical. It's a basic thing: When you work muscles, you damage them. They need time to recover into stronger muscles. The rest of your body—bones, joints, connective tissue—also needs time to repair and recover.

If you don't give your body this time? You'll have overuse injuries, which can be serious. (This is a case of being overmotivated to exercise.)

Think of recovery this way: It's the most important activity you can do when you're not exercising. That's how your body looks at it.

Sleep is job one. In fact, when you're talking about a healthy lifestyle in general, if you had to pick just one area to improve for health, I would say focus on sleep—both the quantity and quality.

SELF-MASSAGE CAN BE MAGICAL

Booking a massage can be indulgent (and healthy). But few of us can get daily or even weekly massages. I recommend self-massage, and the simplest way to do that is with foam rolling. Ten minutes with a foam roller before a workout or while you watch TV at night can help loosen your muscles (including the fascia, a tough material that runs through your muscles) and make them more resilient and cooperative in general.

Quick tip #1: Rolling muscles can be uncomfortable—that generally signals that your muscles need the attention. This discomfort will improve over time if you stick with rolling.

Quick tip #2: If you don't have a foam roller handy, a basketball works in a pinch.

For a useful list of foam roller exercises complete with descriptions, see Part Four.

Why? Good sleep helps you do everything else better. Ever try eating healthy after a lousy night's sleep? Ever want to work out after a lousy night's sleep? Ever been at your best after a lousy night's sleep? Ever been able to fend off cravings for alcohol and other temptations after a lousy night's sleep?

If you give your body time to rest and recover, you'll have an easier time performing and making better choices the next day.

And here's a nice little bonus: Exercising regularly helps you sleep better. Aerobic exercise helps, but resistance training in particular is excellent. In a 2022 study, Iowa State University researchers recruited more than four hundred sedentary and overweight adults.[11] They broke the group into four subsets. One group did cardio exercise for one year, another did resistance exercise for one year, a third group did both, and the last group did nothing.

Exercisers all slept better, but resistance exercisers slept longer with higher quality and less disturbed sleep than the other groups (see Part Four for much more information on the benefits of resistance training).

Above all, respect the ZZZZs.

CHAPTER 14

#10 on "the Big List"

You didn't think we'd forget about #10, did you?

It's a big one. Probably the biggest. That's why I held it back until now.

What do you think? What should it be? Think about all the things that go into your choices. Think in particular about the one annoying, ever-present, intrusive, pain-in-the-butt, and maybe even debilitating thing that holds you back from making better choices.

Any ideas?

I'll give you a hint: You probably don't like to admit it affects you at all.

Okay, here it is . . .

#10 on "the Big List"

1. Biases 2. Perception 3. Incentives 4. Knowledge 5. Curiosity 6. Self-esteem
7. Self-efficacy 8. Control 9. Community **10. Fear**

Yeah. Makes sense now that you see it, right? So let's talk about #10.

Fear Itself

Doesn't fear sum up much of what holds people back from good decisions? Especially when you include it in the context of all the other things you've read in this book, the rest of the Big List in particular.

Fear breeds bias.

Fear distorts perception.

Fear feeds other negative emotions that erode your motivation: anger, sadness, frustration, impatience, defeat, a feeling of futility.

Fear causes you to shrink back, to hide, to obfuscate, to rationalize, to deflect.

Fear of judgment. Fear of the new.

Fear of challenge. Fear of change.

Fear of leaving unhealthy loved ones behind.

Fear of looking ungraceful when starting out.

Fear of discomfort. Fear of effort. Fear of commitment.

Fear of failure.

Fear of success.

Isn't it so wonderfully human that we can fear success and failure at the same time?

Of all the emotions we've talked about affecting our decisions, fear in all its forms must be the most powerful. It rules us in so many ways.

Let's look at just one: fear of failure. A 2022 study of 455 Saudi medical students broke down how "fear of failure" affected people in different—and maybe unsurprising—ways.[1] Women, for example, allowed fear of failure to lower their self-esteem, while men were afraid of being judged negatively by "important others." And these were medical students, who are generally good at pushing themselves to achieve. Fear spares no one.

What about fear of change? Even positive change? That's another big one. Some researchers say fear of change arises from a lack of information and thus a lack of control because we can't predict what will happen when things change. That can certainly apply to, say, a change in management at a big company, but it doesn't really apply here because making positive changes like adding regular physical activity to your life generally produces a *very* predictable outcome: all good. If you fear changes that will bring you a better life, your fear is misplaced.

Data aside, I find that fear of positive changes is linked to fear of success. After all, if you make these changes and do well—awesome, wonderful, stupendous, right? Well, success comes with a type of baggage that scares people. You have to *keep* succeeding, which of course requires a whole lot of continuous work and holds more possibilities of failure. You could backslide and lose all your gains, and people will judge. Or you could keep doing well and wind up distancing yourself from loved ones who don't make the positive changes you do. You could fear that strife, or even loss.

There are other relevant fears with exercise. A friend of mine once worked for a prominent global weight loss brand, and he told me an interesting thing—one I don't think a lot of people consider when they talk about "getting fit" or "exercising more." A majority of people using that system to lose weight found exercising and any related references—such as gyms or images of very fit people—to be intimidating and, for some, exclusionary.

That kind of fear is hard to overcome when you simply don't feel welcome in certain places or under certain circumstances.

Certainly there are ways around that kind of fear—work out at home, start slowly with walking and ramp up over time—but if a person has had a strong negative feeling toward physical activity for that long, it's hard to push past.

So how do you address fear? Is it necessary to eliminate your fears? No. But you do have to find ways to work with them and around them.

Some revealing questions you may want to answer:

- What fears keep me from making healthy choices?
- Why do I perceive these fears as legitimate? What gives them their power?
- What would happen if I ignored them?
- What would happen if I did things that are good for me even though I am intimidated by them?

This book can certainly help, but take debilitating fears seriously. If you can't simply coexist with or work through your fears, I suggest seeking professional help addressing them.

TIME FOR ANOTHER SELF-TEST

Now is a great time to go back and redo the self-test on page 31 in chapter 3. That's the beauty of it—it never gets old or wears out. It simply reflects where you are on the motivational spectrum at any given time, as long as you offer honest answers. Remember, there is no perfection—only improvement, and when you've improved quite a bit, consistency.

Consistency in motivation and action is really all you need.

A Final Thought

A funny thing about all the hang-ups we've discussed in this book: Exercise eliminates most of them. When you're done, all sweaty, winding down, you realize in your bones that a good daily workout unties a lot of knots.

I suggest you go back to page xi and reread Alice's story now that you've read all this other material.

I bet you understand her motivation better now.

I bet, in a way, you find her response to grief and depression unsurprising and maybe even expected. You may even think, *She did what everyone should do.*

That's what I want you to take away from this last bit of the book—that feeling Alice had. No matter your circumstances, you can choose to live the rest of your life under that proverbial black cloud. Or you can tie your sneakers and go out the door.

That's your daily choice.

Either you will or you won't.

I'm rooting for you. And if you ever need some help, I'm right here.

Build Your Own Workouts

NO SUCH THING AS
TOO MANY EXERCISES

I would never say there's an infinite number of exercises in existence, but there's a large enough variety that you have more than enough to do in a lifetime. And yet, a lot of people ask me, "What kind of exercises should I do?" Well, here you go. This section will show you how to build your own basic workouts selected from a variety of exercises. The mission here is simplicity. Workouts don't have to be complex and long to be effective. And these exercises are very effective.

Why did I pick these exercises? The more basic ones are the foundational ones—pushup, squat, lunge, plank—and variations on those. Most people don't need any more than that. But there are more varied and advanced exercises in here as well.

I also include these exercises because they're compound movements, meaning they move more than one joint at a time and hit more muscles all at once. That's functional training and that's efficiency.

The vast majority of these exercises are body weight only, no equipment needed, and can be done anytime/anywhere. I've also added a short section of exercises that include dumbbells (not everyone has 'em, but if you want to add them, you can). Some of those with dumbbells are, again, variations on the basics, because that's all most people need.

The workouts you'll create are of the "Fifty-Word" or less variety: simple, direct, and challenging without requiring much extra aside from remembering which exercises you picked.

Why Do Resistance Workouts?

I've said before that all anyone needs is a nice, brisk walk to get health benefits from exercise. That's true. And I've known folks whose only exercise is running. They're in good shape. And people play team sports, swim, cycle, row, do yoga, take fitness classes, and on and on. But the patients I have who include resistance training (aka strength training) tend to be the ones I see least. Anecdotally, they're the ones who are stronger and less prone to injury when they do all their other active interests. And it's true that a lot more people meet the aerobic exercise guidelines than meet the muscle-strengthening guidelines. Not enough people strength-train.

There's more. Of course, you'll feel stronger and more vital. But I will once again bang my drum: Increasing muscle mass plays a critical role in regulating blood sugar—muscle can help clear glucose from your blood—so those with type 2 diabetes or prediabetes/metabolic syndrome can really benefit from adding muscle. Resistance training also aids metabolic, musculoskeletal, and mental health.[1]

Maintaining muscle is also critical in the aging process, as sarcopenia (muscle loss) and dynapenia (strength loss) accelerate with age and chip away at whatever muscle your body has. A shorter, weaker musclespan/strengthspan leads to shorter healthspan from frailty and a compromised lifespan.

Resistance training remains one of the best antiaging weapons we have.

Then there's the simplest answer of all: You'll be able to do everyday things better. Who doesn't want that?

WHAT'S THE MINIMUM DOSE OF
STRENGTH TRAINING?

A 2022 study in *Research Quarterly for Exercise and Sport* of nearly fifteen thousand people found that strength training once a week, doing single sets of six exercises, brought 30 to 50 percent gains in strength over the first year.[2] That's not a lot of work for a whole lot of gain.

And even if you decide, hey, I'm only going to do strength training because I hate running and cardio and all that nonsense (and that's okay), you will still get long-term health benefits. A 2022 *British Journal of Sports Medicine* study looked at nearly one hundred thousand people over ten years and found that those who engaged in strength training alone had a 9 percent lower risk of all-cause mortality, including cardiovascular risk.[3] So you can enjoy these exercises and do nothing else and gain longevity on top of strength and physical capability.

But if you combine some brisk walking or running with strength training, you might be even better off. The folks in that study who met thresholds for moderate to vigorous aerobic activity enjoyed a 32 percent lower risk of death. But those who added resistance training only one to two times per week to their aerobic work had a 41 percent lower risk.

In terms of motivation, a 2019 *PLOS One* study showed some interesting results.[4] The study split twenty-eight men into two groups. Each group did an identical workout regimen for eight weeks—same frequency, same sets and reps. The difference: One group did the same type of resistance exercises every time. The other group's exercises were randomly assigned; they had no idea what resistance exercises they'd get in any workout.

Both groups had similar strength and muscle-building results. But the guys in the random group showed significant improvement in intrinsic motivation when it came to wanting to work out. So changing up which resistance exercises you do may not increase your results, but it may make you more excited to do them.

WHAT ABOUT FLEXIBILITY?

That's another reason I've picked these exercises. The majority of them contribute to "dynamic flexibility," which is simply flexibility achieved by going through a full range of motion. Static stretching can be helpful—exercises like holding a hamstring stretch for thirty seconds—but I prefer strength training and focusing on full range of motion during those movements. A 2021 review looked at eleven studies involving 452 people and found no difference between stretching and strength training on joint range of motion.[5] The movements in these exercises mimic real-life movements and force your muscles and connective tissue to become better at doing said movements. Many of the exercises also challenge your balance. For most people, that's all you need.

If you want to push your body for more flexibility and balance, I suggest yoga, which can give you an amazing workout and help you feel more connected to how your body moves.

The Fifty-Word Workout Template

The mission: A challenging total-body workout.

This exercise collection is divided into upper-body, lower-body, core, and total-body burner sections.

The basic Fifty-Word Workout template looks like this:

> *Upper body one minute / Rest one minute*
> *Lower body one minute / Rest one minute*
> *Core one minute / Rest one minute*
> *Total-body burner one minute / Rest one minute*
> *Repeat this set three times*

Filling in the template is simple. Pick one upper-body, one lower-body, one core, and one total-body exercise from the group. Boom— instant workout. The exercises I included in those groups guarantee that you'll hit your whole body.

DO YOU NEED HEAVY WEIGHT
TO GET REAL RESULTS?

No. I chose mostly body-weight exercises in this book because you need no or little equipment and they can be done anytime/anyplace. But most important: You can build muscles with or without heavy weights. A study in the *Journal of Strength and Conditioning Research* divided study participants into two groups—one lifting lower weight at higher reps, the other lifting heavier weight at lower reps.[6] Both groups built muscle at similar rates (though the heavy-weight group did see advantages in single-rep max lifts). Point being, your body doesn't know the difference between lifting a twenty-five-pound dumbbell and a percentage of your own body weight. As long as the resistance you use challenges your muscles and you work your muscles almost to failure in each set (while maintaining proper form), you'll get results.

How to Customize for Any Fitness Level

Let's take another look at the template, but this time I'll highlight the areas you can adjust:

> *Upper body* <u>*one*</u> *minute / Rest* <u>*one*</u> *minute*
> *Lower body* <u>*one*</u> *minute / Rest* <u>*one*</u> *minute*
> *Core* <u>*one*</u> *minute / Rest* <u>*one*</u> *minute*
> *Total-body burner* <u>*one*</u> *minute / Rest* <u>*one*</u> *minute*
> *Repeat this set* <u>*three*</u> *times*

See the underlines? That's where you can vary:

- Number of sets
- How much time on each exercise
- How much time you rest

One thing not mentioned in the workout that you can vary: intensity. You determine how hard you go, how long you rest, and how challenging the whole thing will be for you.

You can also vary how many exercises you include. Example: instead of upper body, lower body, core, and total body, maybe starting out you just do two different total-body exercises and that's it. Or maybe you want to have an upper-body day and do two or three upper exercises. Same goes for lower-body day. And you can add even more exercises to make the workout longer and more challenging.

You can vary the order of everything as well. Start with core, or lower body, or whichever you choose.

That's it. That's how easy it is to build a simple, effective workout.

What Does "Warm-Up" Really Mean?

You should always warm up before a workout. I suggest a five- to ten-minute preworkout session to prepare your body for the work it's about to do. I've used the analogy of a frozen rubber band—you give it a yank and it will snap. That's your muscles without a warm-up. You want your "rubber bands" to be warm and flexible before you stress them. What qualifies as "warm"? Basically, you want to have raised your heart rate and broken a light sweat before you start your main session. How to do this? Here's a circuit to run through that can do the job. Perform each for thirty seconds or do ten to twenty reps depending on your fitness level before you begin your regular workout.

JUMPING JACKS
Stand with your feet together and your hands at your sides. Simultaneously raise your extended arms above your head and jump up just enough to spread your feet out wide. Without pausing, quickly reverse the movement and repeat. Keep your ankles locked by pulling your toes up, and bounce on the balls of your feet.

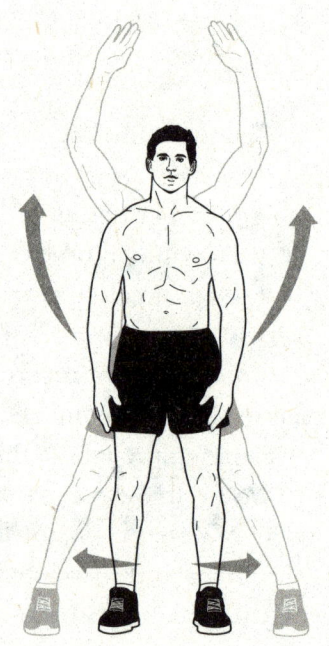

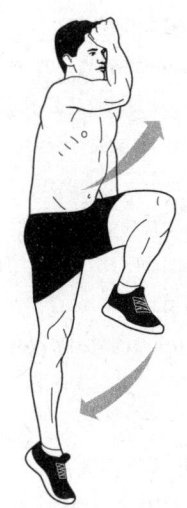

WALKING HIGH KNEES

Stand tall with your feet shoulder-width apart. Without changing your posture, raise your right knee as high as you can and step forward. Repeat with your left leg. Continue to alternate back and forth.

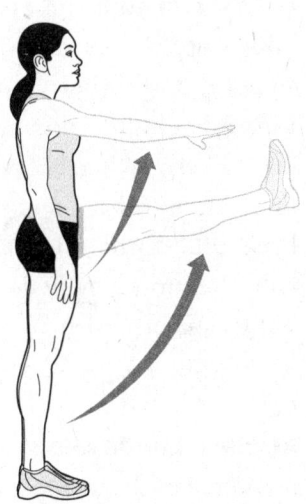

WALKING HIGH KICKS

Stand tall with your hands hanging at your sides. Keeping your knee straight, kick your left leg up—reaching with your right arm out to meet it—as you simultaneously take a step forward (just imagine you're a Russian soldier). As soon as your left foot touches the ground, repeat the movement with your right leg and left arm. Alternate back and forth.

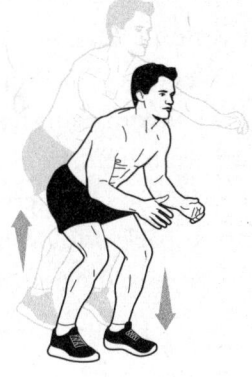

POGO HOP

Stand in an athletic stance with your feet hip-width apart and your arms bent around ninety degrees. Keeping your body upright, repeatedly jump up, allowing your feet to move only a few inches from the floor. Keep your ankles locked, toes flexed up, and foot contact on the balls of your feet.

GATE SWING

Stand with your feet together and your hands at your sides. Drop into a squat by pushing your hips back and lower your body toward the floor while keeping your back upright. Make sure your toes point outward, and gently press your hands on your inner thighs to open your knees as far as you can to facilitate the stretch. Hop back to start position and repeat.

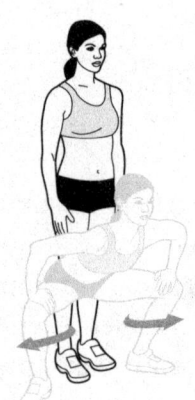

HIP SWING

Stand tall and hold on to a sturdy object with your right hand. Brace your core. Keep your right knee straight, and swing your right leg forward as high as you comfortably can. Then, swing backward as far as you can. That's one rep. Swing back and forth continuously for half the time, then do the same with your other leg.

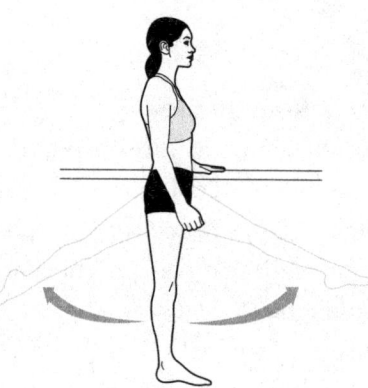

REVERSE LUNGE AND REACH-BACK

Stand tall with your feet hip-width apart. Step backward with your right leg, and lower your body until your left knee is bent at least ninety degrees. Once in this position, reach your arms up and back toward your left shoulder. Press back up to a standing position, and then step back with your left leg, this time reaching toward your right.

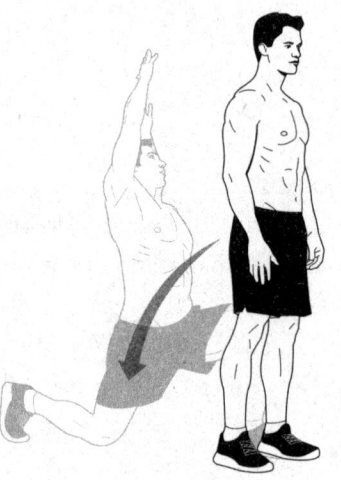

INCHWORMS

Stand tall with your legs straight, and bend over and touch the floor. Keeping your legs straight, walk your hands forward as far as you can without letting your hips sag. Then, take tiny steps to walk your feet back to your hands. That's one repetition.

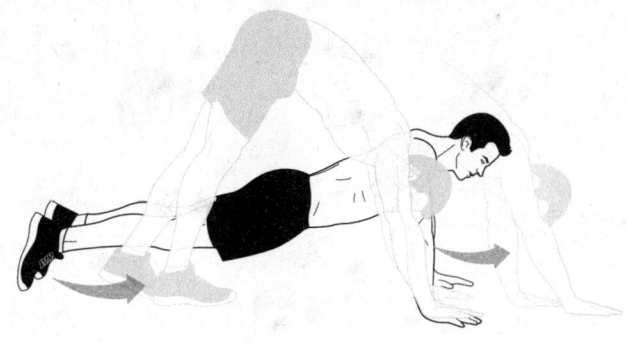

The Exercises

Upper Body

PUSHUP

Get down on all fours, placing your hands slightly wider than your shoulders. Straighten your arms and legs. Lower your body until your chest nearly touches the floor. Pause, and push yourself back up. Repeat for the allotted time.

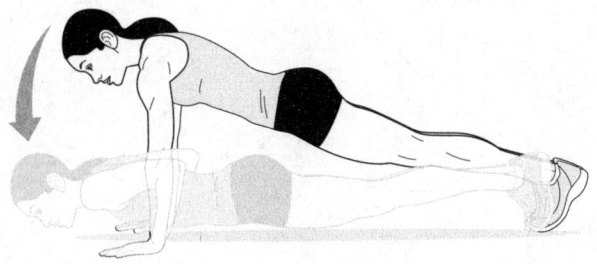

CLOSE-HANDS PUSHUP

Assume a standard pushup position (your body should form a straight line from your ankles to your head). Brace your abs, squeeze your glutes, and keep your elbows tucked in against your sides as you lower yourself until your chest is about an inch from the floor. Pause and push up to starting position.

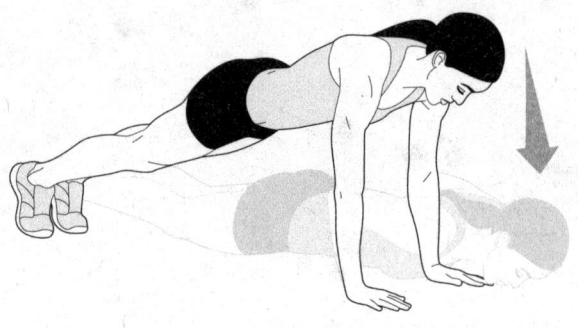

PLYO PUSHUP

Assume a pushup position with your hands slightly beyond shoulder-width and your body in a straight line from head to ankles. Bend your elbows and lower your body until your chest nearly touches the floor; then push up with enough force that your hands leave the 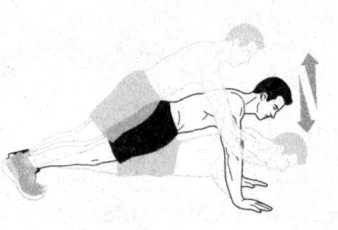 floor. Note: Control your motion to soften the landing on your wrists to prevent injury. To make this exercise easier, elevate your hands on a step, bench, or box.

PUSHBACK PUSHUP

Assume a pushup position with your arms straight and hands slightly wider than your shoulders. Bend at the elbows and lower your torso until your chest nearly touches the floor. Pause, then push your butt toward your ankles until your knees are bent ninety degrees. Return to the starting position and repeat.

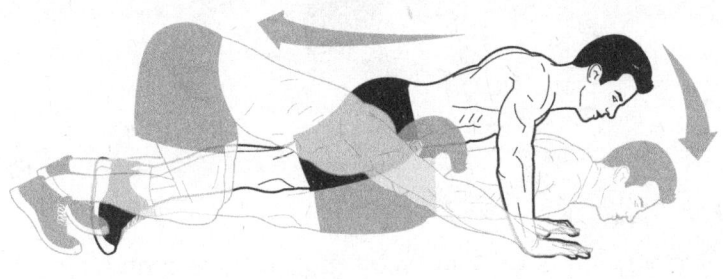

CHANGE-UP PUSHUP

Assume a pushup position with your hands together. Do a pushup. Place your hands shoulder-width apart. Do a pushup. Spread your hands to twice shoulder-width and do a pushup. Continue reps back to close-hands and repeat cycle for the allotted time.

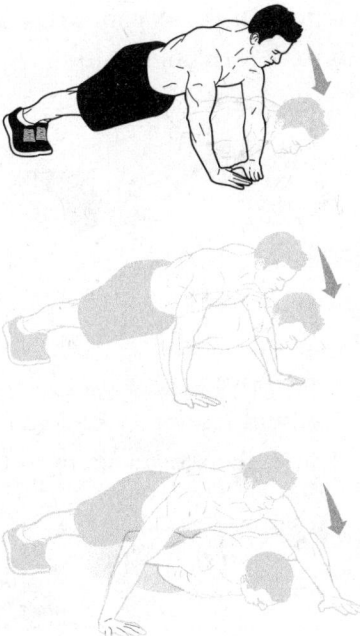

SINGLE-LEG PUSHUP

Assume a pushup position. While descending, lift your right leg eight to ten inches off the floor. Return to the starting position and descend again, this time raising your left leg. Alternate for the allotted time.

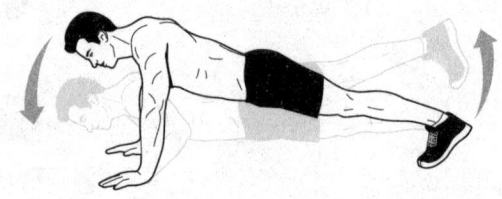

FLOOR Y-T-I RAISES

Note: Do one rep of each and start again at the beginning for the allotted time.

Lie face down and allow your arms to rest on the floor, completely straight and at a thirty-degree angle to your body, your palms facing each other and your thumbs up (your body should resemble the letter Y). Raise your arms as high as you can, pause, then lower them to the starting position.

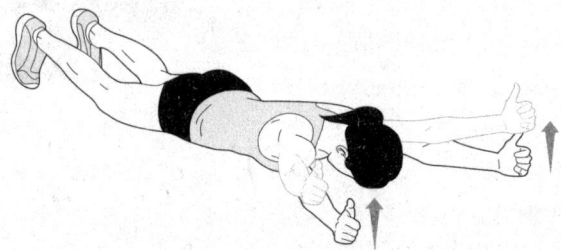

Now move your arms so they are straight out to your sides (your body should resemble the letter T). Raise your arms as high as you can, pause, then lower them to the starting position.

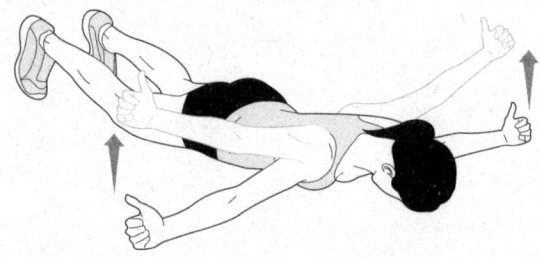

Now position your arms so they're straight above your shoulders (your body should resemble the letter I). Raise your arms as high as you can, pause, then lower them to the starting position.

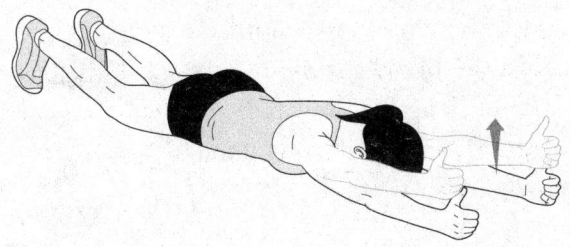

BENCH DIP

Sit on a flat bench with your hands on the bench at your sides (or grip the sides of a chair seat). Keep your palms on the bench at all times with your fingers facing forward and your palms down. Walk your feet out a couple of steps until your legs are extended, and lower your body down just in front of the bench until your 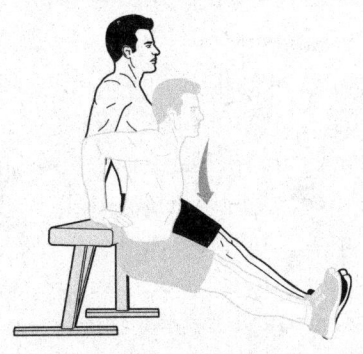 elbows are at ninety degrees. Then press through your palms to raise your body. For a bigger challenge, put your feet up on another bench/chair so your legs are horizontal to the floor.

INVERTED SHOULDER PRESS

Assume the pushup position with your feet on a bench or chair, and push your hips up so your torso is nearly perpendicular to the floor. Your hands should be slightly wider than your shoulders, and your arms straight. Without changing your body posture, lower yourself until your head nearly touches the floor. Pause, then return to the starting position.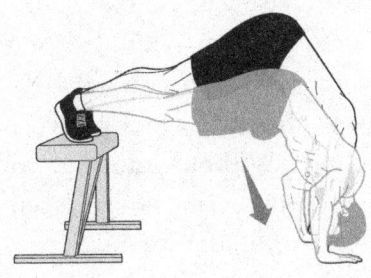

Upper-Body Dumbbell Variations

DUMBBELL ROW

Holding two dumbbells, bend at your hips
and knees and lower your torso until it's
nearly parallel to the floor. Let the dumbbells hang at arm's length. Now pull the
dumbbells up to the sides of your chest.
Pause, and slowly lower them.

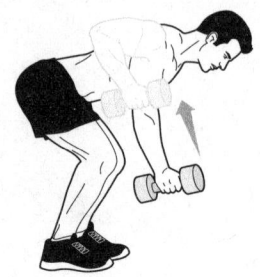

DUMBBELL PUSHUP TO ROW

Assume pushup position with
a dumbbell gripped in each
hand as your base. Lower your
body and perform one pushup.
Now pull the right dumbbell
up to the side of your chest.
Pause, then lower it and repeat
with the left side. That's one
rep. Perform as many as you
can in the allotted time.

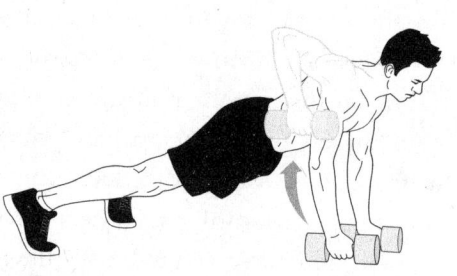

REAR LATERAL RAISE

Grab a pair of dumbbells and bend forward at your hips until your torso is
nearly parallel to the floor. Set your
feet shoulder-width apart. Let the
dumbbells hang straight down from
your shoulders, your palms facing each
other. Without moving your torso,
raise your arms straight out to your
sides until they're in line with your
body. Pause, then slowly return to the
starting position.

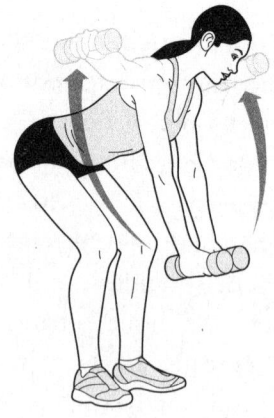

ALTERNATING DUMBBELL CURL AND PRESS

Stand with a pair of dumbbells just outside your shoulders, arms bent, palms facing each other. Press the left dumbbell overhead as you lower the right one to your side. Reverse the move as you return to the start; then press the right dumbbell overhead and lower the left. Alternate for the allotted time.

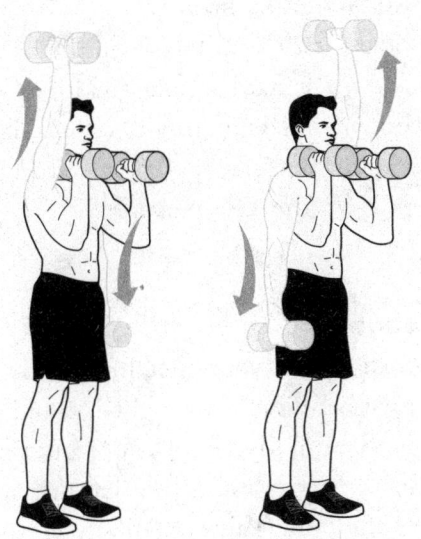

PUSHUP-POSITION HAMMER CURL

Grip a pair of dumbbells and assume a pushup position with your palms facing each other. Brace your core and glutes. Without moving your upper arm, curl the weight in your right hand toward your right shoulder. Lower it and repeat with your left arm. Alternate for the allotted time.

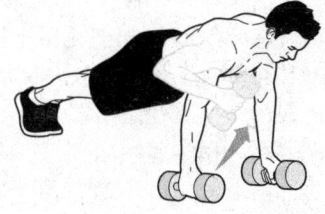

Lower Body

BODY-WEIGHT SQUAT

Stand with your hands on the back of your head and your feet shoulder-width apart. Lower your body until your thighs are parallel to the floor. Pause, then return to the starting position. Repeat for the allotted time.

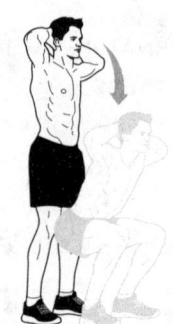

LUNGE

Stand with your feet hip-width apart. Step forward with your right leg and lower your body until the top of your right thigh is parallel to the floor and your left knee comes close to the floor. Pause, then return to the starting position. Alternate legs for the allotted time.

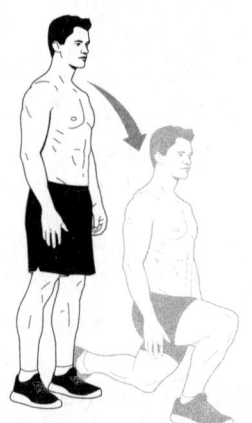

WALKING LUNGE

Stand with your feet hip-width apart. Step forward with your right leg and lower your body until the top of your right thigh is parallel to the floor and your left knee comes close to the floor. Without rising, lunge forward with your left leg. Keep your torso upright and swing your arms in a running motion with each lunge. Alternate legs for half the allotted time, then perform reverse lunges back to the starting point.

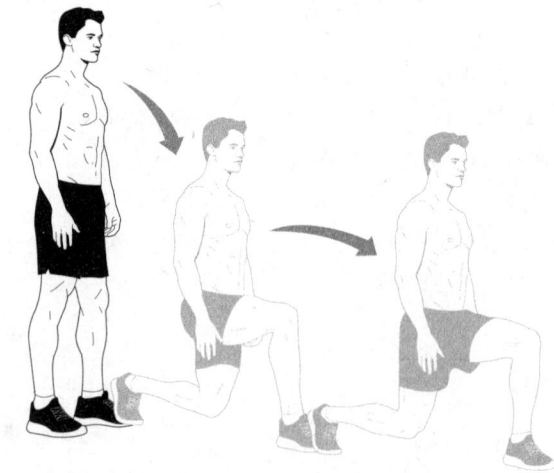

MULTIDIRECTIONAL HOP

Stand with your knees slightly bent. Jump forward twelve inches and land on your right foot. Hop backward to the start, landing on both feet. Repeat on your left foot. Next, do the sequence going sideways. Continue through the allotted time. (Hold a dumbbell in front of your chest with both hands for an added challenge.)

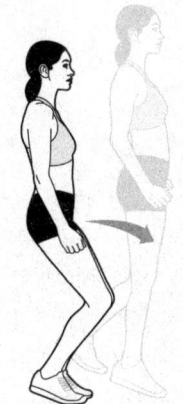

SKATER HOP

This exercise mimics the explosive side-to-side movements of speed skaters. Stand on your right foot with your right knee slightly bent and place your left foot back and behind your right ankle. Bend your right knee and lower your body into a partial squat. Then explosively bound to the left by jumping off your right foot. Land on your left foot and bring your right foot back, behind, and across your left leg. Reach your right hand toward your left foot. Move back to the right, landing on your right foot and touching the ground with your left hand. Repeat alternating sides.

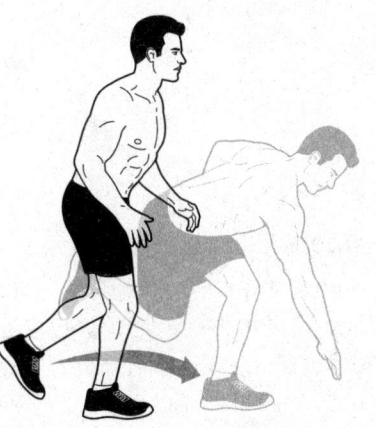

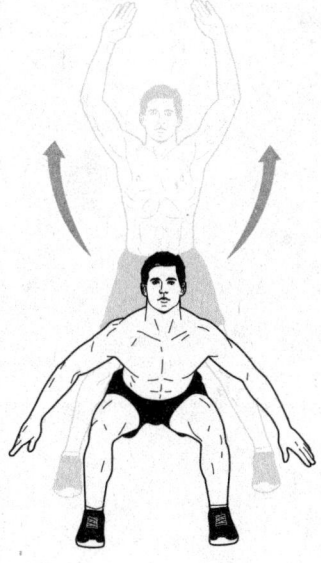

STAR JUMP

With feet about shoulder-width apart, squat down so your hands move down to the ground near your feet. Then, in one movement, jump up into the air and spread your arms and legs as wide as you possibly can. Return to starting position and repeat.

SQUAT JUMP

Start with your feet shoulder-width apart and hands on hips. Now squat with your heels flat and touch the ground with your palms. Jump force-fully, thrusting your arms overhead with palms inward to boost momentum. Land and immediately begin the next jump.

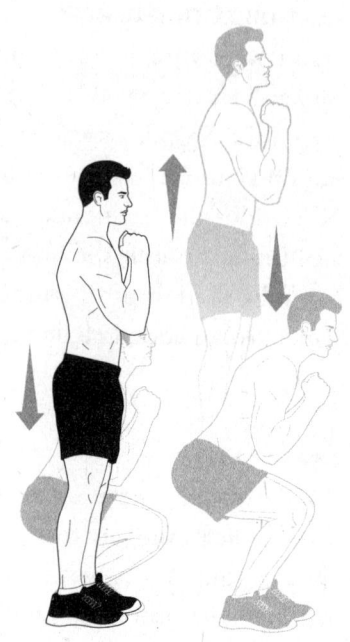

SINGLE-LEG DEADLIFT REACH

Stand and raise your left foot and left hand. Slowly lower your torso and touch the toes of your right foot with your left hand. Return to the starting position. Work for half the allotted time and switch sides.

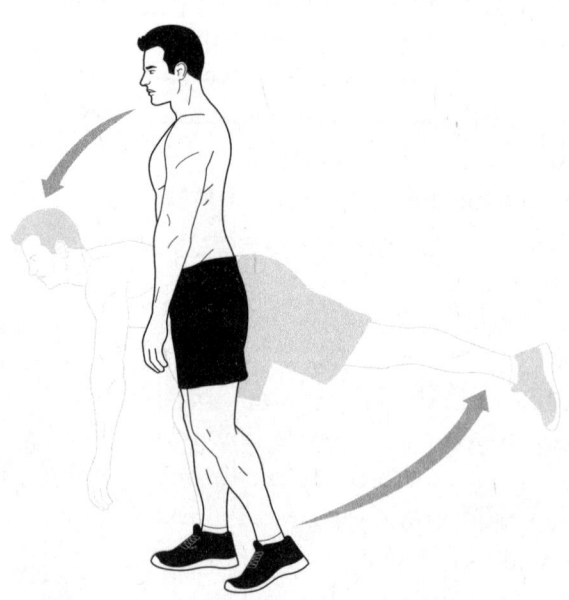

COMPASS LUNGE

Stand with your feet hip-width apart. Step forward (or "north") with your right leg and lower your body until the top of your right thigh is parallel to the floor and your left knee comes close to the floor. Push back to standing and repeat the exercise while hitting points on the compass (northeast, east, etc.). Note: Northern

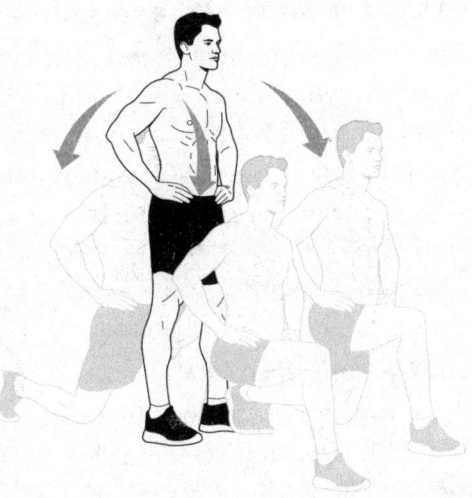

lunges are forward, southern are reverse, east and west are side lunges. When you hit "due south," switch legs and continue until you reach north again. Do as much as you can in the allotted time.

LOW SIDE-TO-SIDE LUNGE

Stand with your feet shoulder-width apart and facing straight ahead. Clasp your hands in front of your chest (or use dumbbells as illustrated). Shift your weight to your right leg and lower your body, bending your right knee and pushing your butt back. Keep your left leg straight and left foot flat on the floor. Without raising yourself all the way to standing, shift the movement to the left. Alternate back and forth. Note: Be sure to push your hips back as you lower down, and engage your core to keep your upper body vertical.

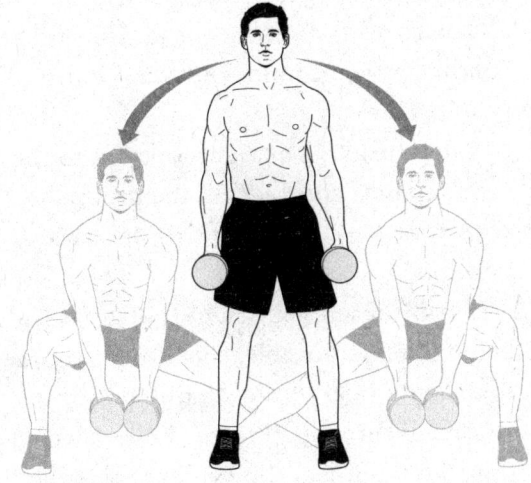

REVERSE LUNGE WITH TOE TOUCH

Stand with your feet hip-width apart. Step back with your right leg and lower your body until your knee almost touches the floor. Stand up, swing your right leg as high as you can, and touch your toes with your left hand. Alternate sides for the allotted time.

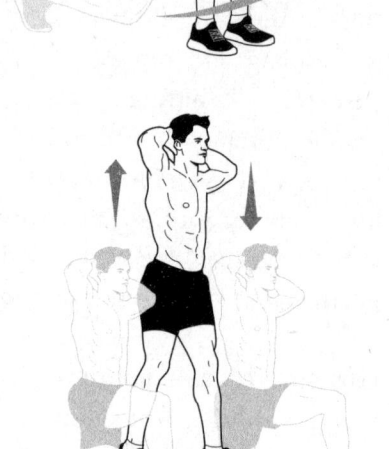

BODY-WEIGHT SPLIT JUMP

Place your hands on your hips and assume a staggered stance, left leg forward. Slowly lower your body as far as you can, and then jump with enough force to propel both feet off the floor. Land with your right leg forward. That's one rep. Alternate back and forth for the allotted time.

THREE-POINT BALANCE TOUCH

Standing on your left leg with your knee slightly bent and chest up, perform a quarter squat. Your right leg (nonbalancing leg) will have three actions without anything else moving:

a. Reach your right foot as far forward as possible and gently tap the ground, and then return to starting position.

b. Next, reach your right foot out to the right as far as possible, tap the ground with your toes, and return to the starting position.

c. Finally, reach your right foot as far back behind you as possible, touch with your toes, and return to the starting position.

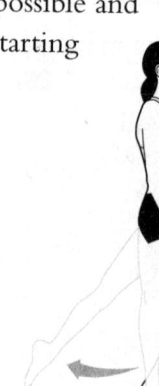

That's one repetition. The deeper you squat your left leg, the harder it becomes.

FROG JUMP

Squat and touch the ground with both hands, keeping your arms straight. Then explode into the air, raising your knees as high as they'll go.

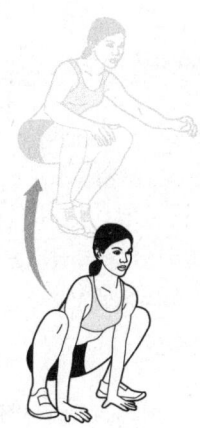

SUMO BURPEE

Stand with your feet several inches wider than your shoulders, then squat (resembling a squatting sumo wrestler) and place your hands on the floor in front of you. Kick your legs back into a pushup position, quickly bring your legs back to a squat, and jump up, throwing your hands above your head. Land and repeat.

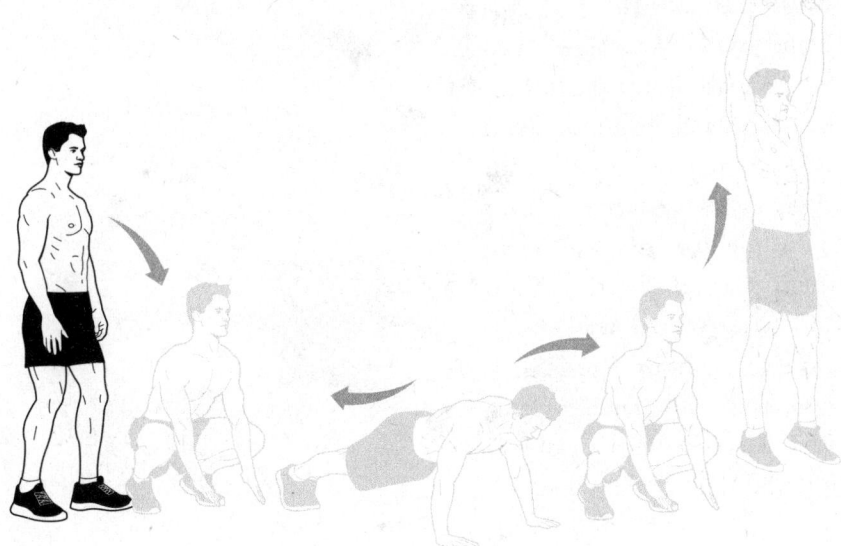

Lower-Body Dumbbell Variations

DUMBBELL SQUAT

Stand with your feet shoulder-width apart, holding a dumbbell in each hand at your sides. Lower your body until your thighs are parallel to the floor. Pause, then return to the starting position. Repeat for the allotted time.

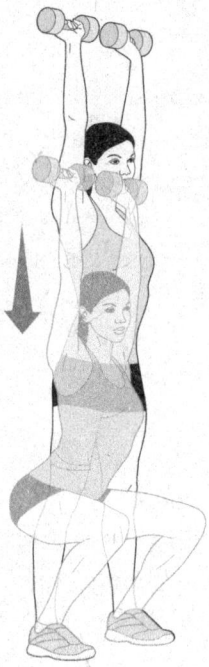

DUMBBELL LUNGE

Stand with your feet hip-width apart, holding a dumbbell in each hand at your sides. Step forward with your right leg and lower your body until the top of your right thigh is parallel to the floor and your left knee comes close to the floor. Pause, then return to the starting position. Alternate legs for the allotted time.

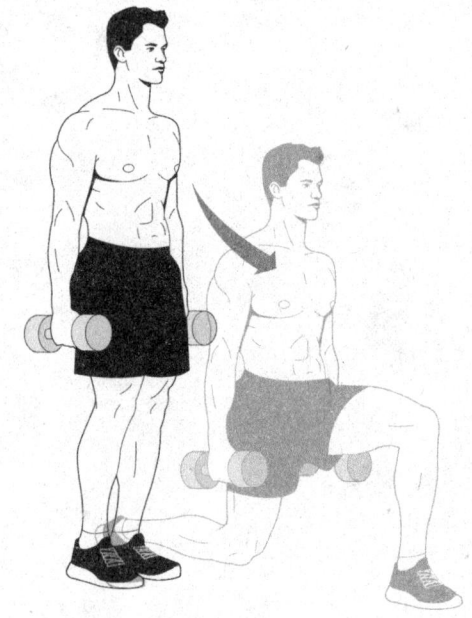

DUMBBELL BULGARIAN SPLIT SQUAT

Hold a pair of dumbbells at arm's length next to your hips. Stand in a staggered stance and place the top of your back foot on a bench, step, or chair. Keeping your torso upright, bend your front knee and lower your body as far as you can. Pause, and push back to the start. Halfway through the allotted time, switch legs.

DUMBBELL STEP-UP

Grab a pair of dumbbells and hold them at arm's length at your sides. Stand facing a bench or step and place your left foot on it. Press your left heel into the bench and push your body up until your left leg is straight and you're standing on one leg. (Keep your right foot elevated.) Now lower your body until your right foot touches the floor. That's one rep. Repeat for half the allotted time, then switch legs.

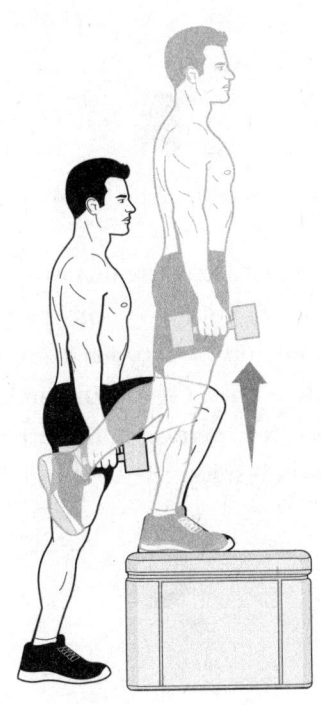

Core

PLANK

Assume a pushup position but with your weight on your forearms. Brace your abs, clench your glutes, and keep your body straight from head to heel.

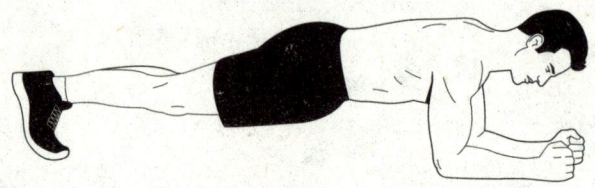

SIDE PLANK

Lie on your right side, prop yourself up on your right forearm, and raise your hips so your body is straight from ankles to head. Hold for half the allotted time, then switch sides and repeat.

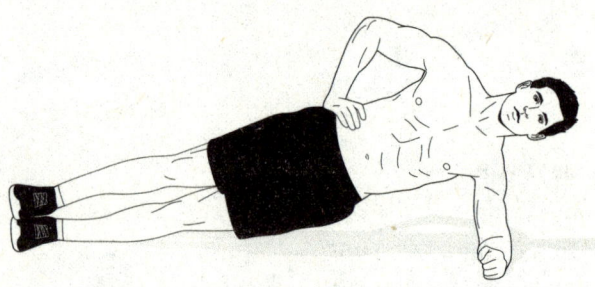

SINGLE-LEG SIDE PLANK

Lie on your side and use your forearm to support your body. Raise your hips until your body forms a straight line from shoulder to ankles. Then raise your top leg as high as you can and hold it that way for the duration of the exercise. Halfway through the prescribed time, switch sides.

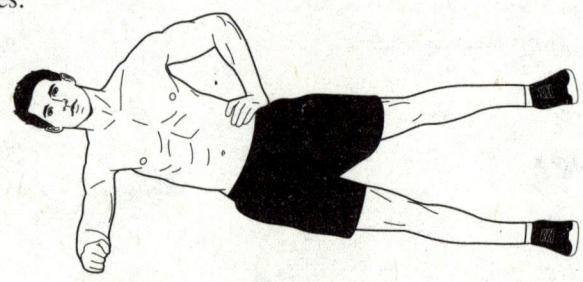

SINGLE-LEG, SINGLE-ARM PLANK

Assume a pushup position but with your weight on your forearms. Brace your abs, clench your glutes, and keep your body straight from head to heel. Raise your right leg and hold it for five seconds. Then lower it and raise your left leg for five seconds. Alternate legs for the allotted time.

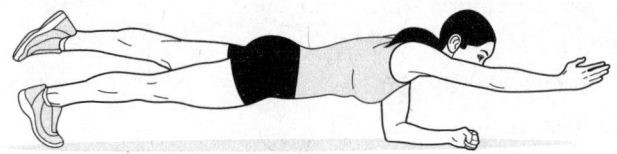

HIP RAISE

Lie face up on the floor with your knees bent and your feet flat on the floor. Raise your hips so your body forms a straight line from your shoulders to your knees. Clench your glutes as you reach the top of the movement. Pause, and then lower your body back to the starting position.

ELEVATED BIRD DOG

Assume a pushup position and "walk" your feet forward so your knees are bent about ninety degrees and slightly above the floor. Raise your right arm and left leg until they're in line with your body. Return to the starting position, and then repeat with your left arm and right leg. Alternate arms and legs with each rep.

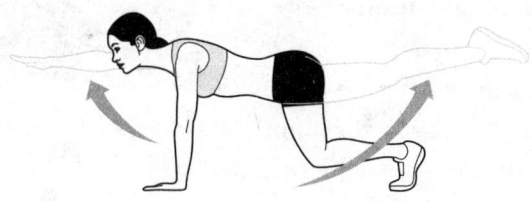

BICYCLE CRUNCH

Lie face up with your hips and knees bent ninety degrees so that your lower legs are parallel to the floor. Place your fingers on the sides of your forehead. Lift your shoulders off the floor and hold them there. Twist your upper body to the right as you pull your right knee in as fast as you can until it touches your left elbow. Simultaneously straighten your left leg. Return to the starting position and repeat to the other side.

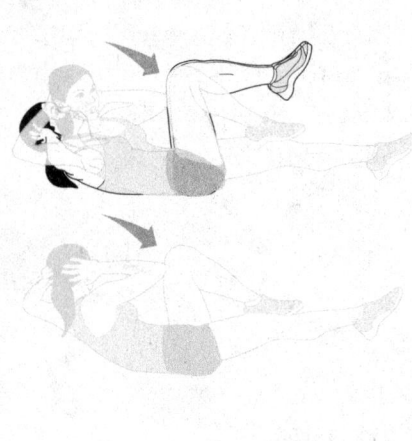

THREE-POINT CORE TOUCH

Assume a pushup position. Now quickly move your right leg forward so your right heel lands outside your right hand. Pause and return to the pushup position. Now quickly move your right leg forward so your right foot lands outside your left hand, and then return to the pushup position. That's one rep. Work for half the allotted time and repeat with your left leg.

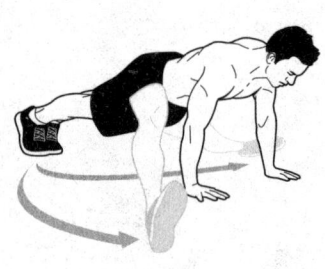

HIP-UP

Lie on your left side, right arm extended so it's perpendicular to the floor. Prop yourself up on your left forearm and raise your hips so your body is straight from ankles to head. Lower your left hip, and then raise it again until it's in line with your body. Halfway through the allotted time, switch and repeat on your right side.

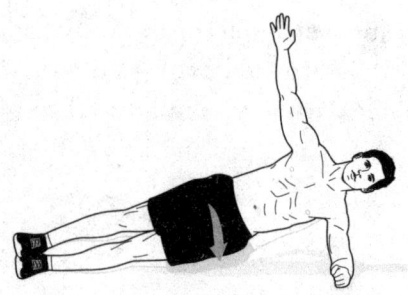

LEG TUCK AND TWIST

Sit and lean back forty-five degrees, your legs straight and palms on the floor behind you. Lift your legs off the floor. Pull your knees toward your left shoulder as you twist your torso to your left. Return to the starting position and repeat to your right.

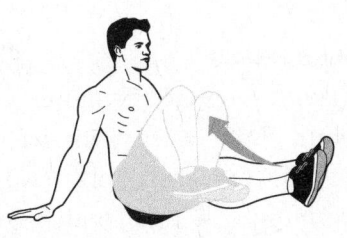

SINGLE-LEG HIP RAISE

Lie on your back with your right foot flat and your left leg raised so it's in line with your right thigh. Push your hips up, keeping your left leg elevated. Pause and slowly return to the starting position. Switch legs halfway through the allotted time.

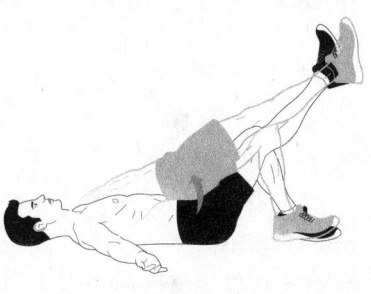

PRONE COBRA

Lie on the floor with your legs straight and your arms at your sides, palms down. Contract your glutes and lift your head, chest, arms, and legs off the floor. Simultaneously rotate your

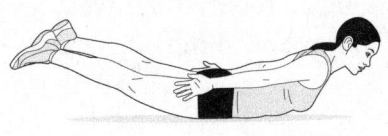

arms so your thumbs point toward the ceiling. Your hips should be the only part of your body touching the floor. Hold for a five-count and return to start. Perform as many as you can in the allotted time.

FIGURE EIGHT

Lie on your back with your arms at your sides, palms down. Raise your legs so they form a forty-five-degree angle with the floor. Now make big, looping circles with your legs, first to your right and then to your left, forming a sideways figure eight. That's one rep.

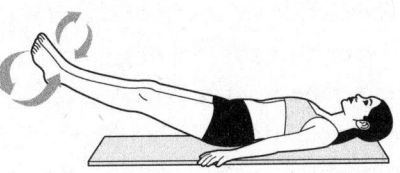

Total-Body Burners

HIGH KNEES

Sprint in place, bringing your knees up to your chest. Keep your back straight as you pump your arms and drive your hands past your hips in time with your legs. Alternate knees for the allotted time. Note: If you have room, such as working outdoors, substitute regular running sprints.

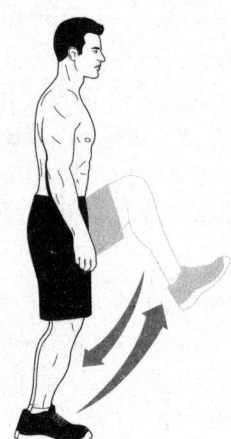

SHUTTLE RUN

Set up two cones or other kind of markers ten to twenty-five yards apart (depending on how much room you have). Sprint from one to the other and back.

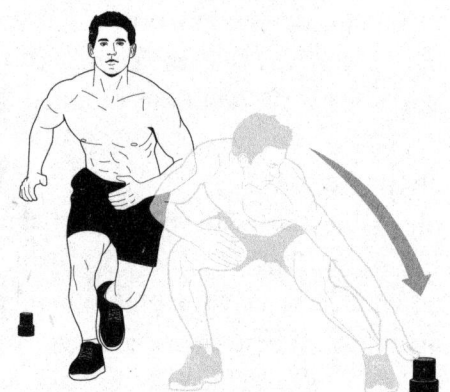

MOUNTAIN CLIMBER

Assume a pushup position. Your body should form a straight line from your head to your ankles. Without allowing your lower-back posture to change, lift your left foot off the floor and move your left knee toward your chest. Return to the starting position, and repeat with your right leg. Alternate the move with each leg quickly.

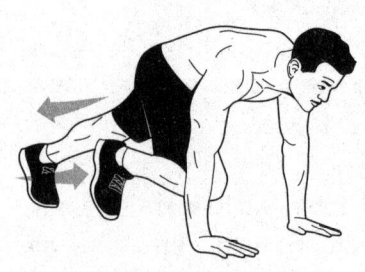

BURPEE

Stand with your feet shoulder-width apart. Squat as deeply as you can and place your hands on the floor. Kick into a pushup position. Bring your legs back to a squat and jump up, throwing your hands above your head. Land and repeat.

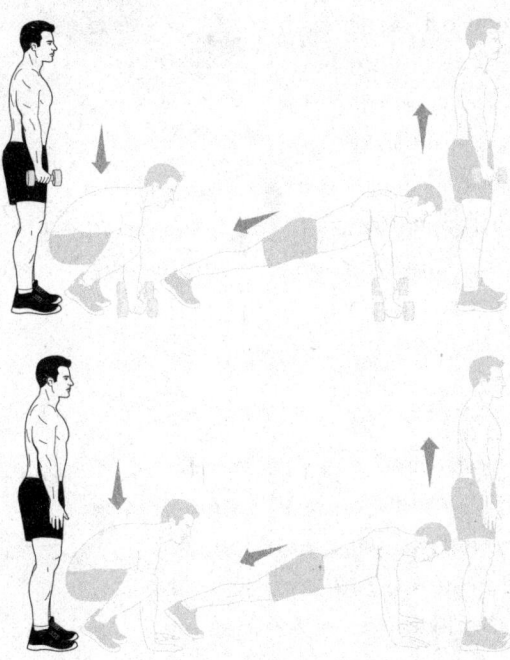

BURPEE WITH PUSHUP

Stand with your feet shoulder-width apart. Squat as deeply as you can and place your hands on the floor. Kick back into a pushup position. Do one pushup. Bring your legs back to a squat and jump up, throwing your hands above your head. Land and repeat.

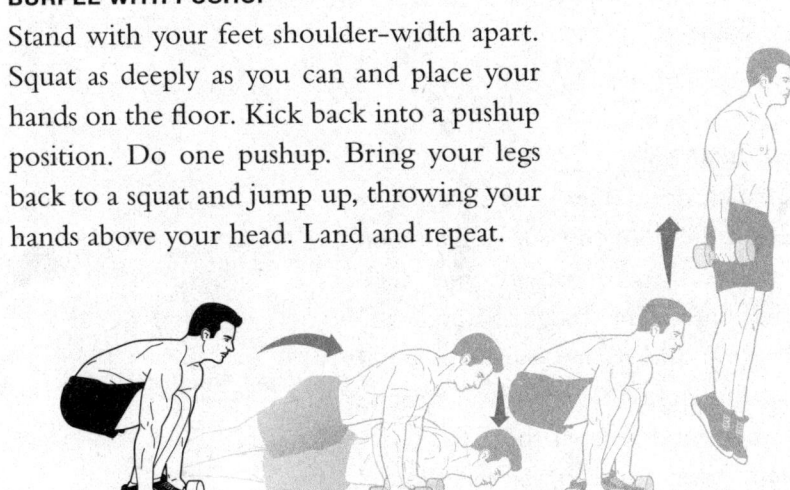

LIZARD CRAWL

Position your body on the floor in pushup position. Walk forward with your right arm as you simultaneously lift your left foot up and step forward. With each step you should lower your body toward the floor. Continue this alternating action, as if you are crawling, but your knees are off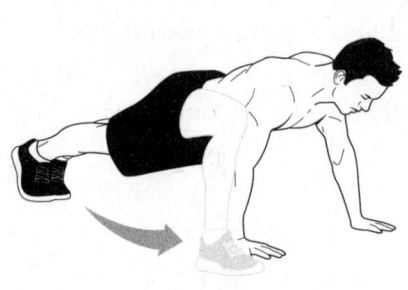

the ground. With each step of your foot, your knee will come close to touching your elbow. Your back should stay straight throughout the range of motion.

CRAB ROLL

Sit with your palms and feet on the floor. Raise your hips so your body is a straight line from your knees to your shoulders; this is the starting position. Lift your left foot and right hand and flip over to your left, placing your right hand back on the floor and kicking your left leg out behind you. (Keep it elevated.) Flip back to the start. That's one rep.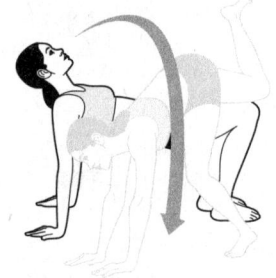

MOGUL JUMP

Get on all fours and lift your knees a few inches off the floor so your weight is on your hands and the balls of your feet. Keeping your arms straight and legs together, hop and rotate your knees and feet to the right. Now hop and rotate your knees and feet to the left. That's one rep. Alternate sides for the allotted time.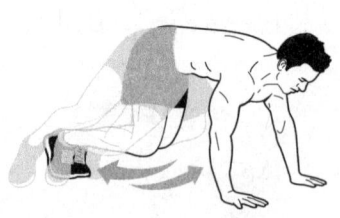

Total-Body Dumbbell Variations

DUMBBELL SWING

(Note: You can also use a kettlebell for this exercise.) Using both hands, hold a dumbbell by one end with your arms hanging straight down in front of you. Stand with your feet hip-width apart, chest up, shoulders back. Bend your knees slightly and push the weight back between your legs, then explode forward and upward with your hips to propel the weight out in front of you. Brace your core and squeeze your glutes as you swing the weight up using momentum until the weight is at chest height. In a smooth motion, swing the weight back down between your legs and repeat.

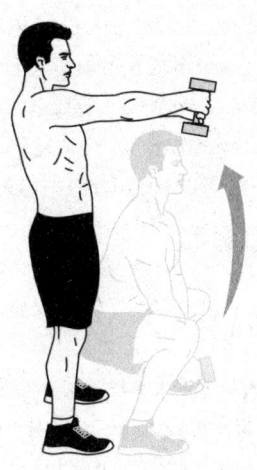

DUMBBELL SKIER SWING

Holding a pair of dumbbells at arm's length next to your sides, stand with your feet hip-width apart and your knees slightly bent. Without rounding your lower back, bend at your hips as you simultaneously swing your arms backward. Now explosively thrust your hips forward and raise your torso until you're standing upright while allowing your momentum to swing the weights up to chest level. (Don't actively lift the weight.) Swing back and forth for the allotted time.

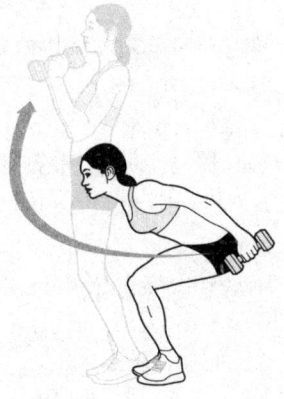

DUMBBELL CHOP

Hold a dumbbell with both hands above your right shoulder. Stand with your feet shoulder-width apart. Brace your core and rotate your torso to the right. While keeping your arms straight, swing the dumbbell down and to the outside of your left knee by rotating to the left and bending at your hips. Reverse the movement to return to the start. Halfway through the prescribed time, switch sides.

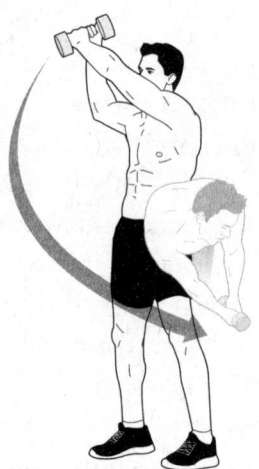

DUMBBELL STRAIGHT-LEG DEADLIFT

Hold a pair of dumbbells in front of your thighs with your feet hip-width apart and your knees slightly bent. Hinge forward at your hips, lowering your torso until it's nearly parallel to the floor. Pause, and return to the starting position.

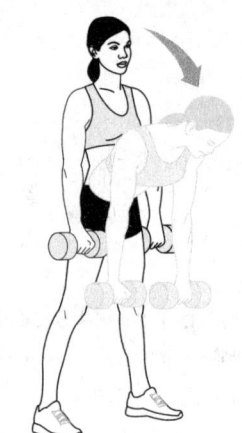

SINGLE-LEG DUMBBELL DEADLIFT

Grab a pair of dumbbells and stand on your left foot. Lift your right foot behind you and bend your knees so your right lower leg is parallel to the floor. Bend forward at your hips and slowly lower your body as far as you can, or until your right lower leg almost touches the floor. Pause, then push your body back to the starting position. Halfway through the prescribed time, switch legs.

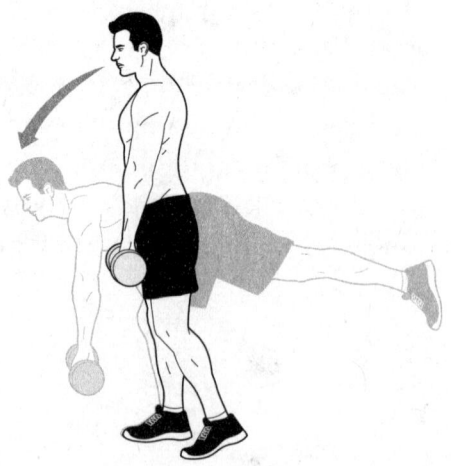

FARMER'S CARRY

Grab a pair of heavy dumbbells and let them hang naturally at arm's length by your sides, holding them as tightly as possible. Now walk for as long as you can before your grip starts to fail. (Forward and backward in equal time; for an added challenge, walk on your toes to target your calves.) If you can walk for longer than sixty seconds, you're ready for a heavier weight.

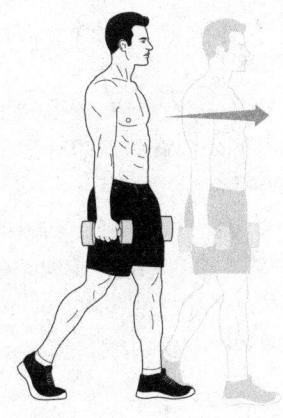

WAITER'S WALK

Stand straight and raise a dumbbell over your head with your right hand (like a waiter carrying a tray). Now walk forward and backward (you can mix it up). Shift the weight to your opposite hand halfway through the allotted time. If you can walk for longer than sixty seconds, use a heavier dumbbell.

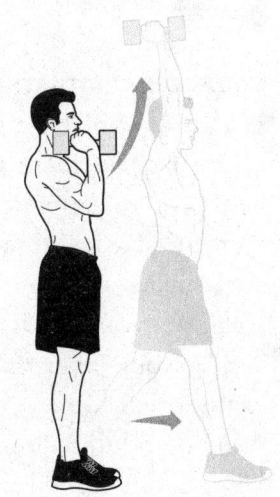

TURKISH GET-UP

Lie with your left leg bent, right arm by your side, and a dumbbell or kettlebell in your left hand above your chest. Now roll onto your right side, prop up on your right forearm, and push yourself into a half kneel by threading your right leg behind your left. Stand up to complete the move. Reverse it to return to the starting position. Switch sides halfway through the allotted time.

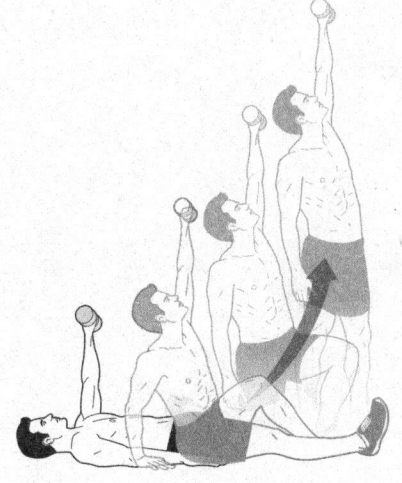

SPLIT-JACK CURL

Hold a pair of dumbbells at your sides, palms in, feet hip-width apart. Jump into a split stance—left leg forward—while curling the weights to your shoulders. Return to the starting position and repeat, landing with your right leg forward. Alternate for the allotted time.

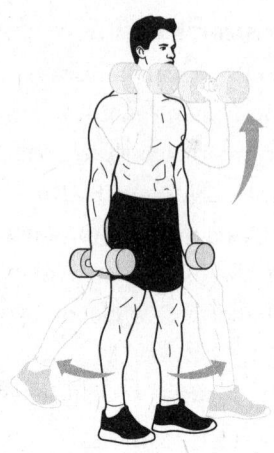

SQUAT CONCENTRATION CURL

Hold a pair of light dumbbells and stand with your feet about shoulder-width apart and your toes pointed out slightly. Push your hips back and squat until your thighs are parallel to the floor. Keeping your weight on your heels, your elbows pressed against your inner thighs, and your palms facing each other, curl and lower the weights for the allotted time. Do it one arm at a time to add an element of instability and increase the challenge to your core.

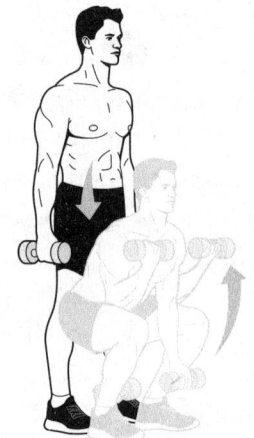

Foam Rolling

FOAM ROLL GLUTES

Sit on a foam roller, with it positioned on your right glute. Cross your right leg over the front of your left thigh. Put your hands on the floor for support. Roll your body forward and backward in small movements from your lower glute to your upper glute. Repeat with the roller under your left glute.

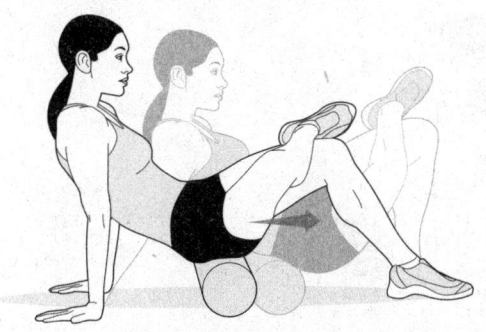

FOAM ROLL ILIOTIBIAL BAND (IT BAND)

Lie on your left side and place your left hip on a foam roller. Put your hands on the floor for support. Cross your right leg over your left, and place your right foot flat on the floor. Roll your body forward and backward in small movements until the roller reaches just above your knee. Repeat on other side.

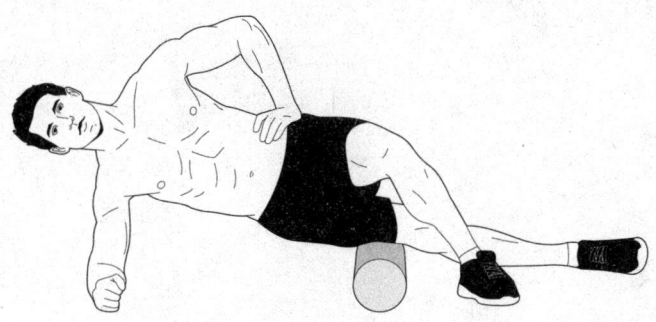

FOAM ROLL CALVES

Sit on the floor and stretch your legs out in front of your body. Place a foam roller under your right calf with your right leg straight. Cross your left leg over your right ankle. Put your hands flat on the floor for support, and raise your body off the floor while keeping your back naturally arched. Roll your body forward until the roller has crossed your entire calf region. Roll back and forth. Repeat with the roller under your left calf.

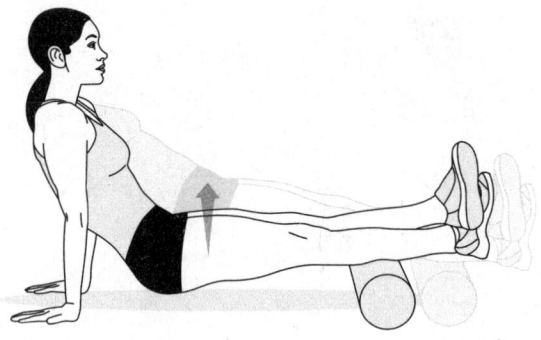

FOAM ROLL QUADS

Lie face down on the floor with a foam roller positioned below both of your knees. Slowly roll your body back and forth over the roller until it reaches the tops of your thighs. Roll back and forth.

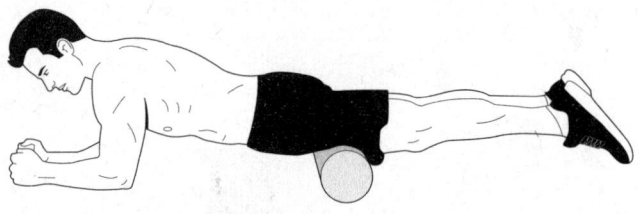

FOAM ROLL HAMSTRINGS

Sit on a foam roller with it positioned just below your right glute, at the top of your right hamstring. Put your hands on the floor for support. Roll your body forward and backward along the length of your hamstring. Repeat with the roller under your left hamstring.

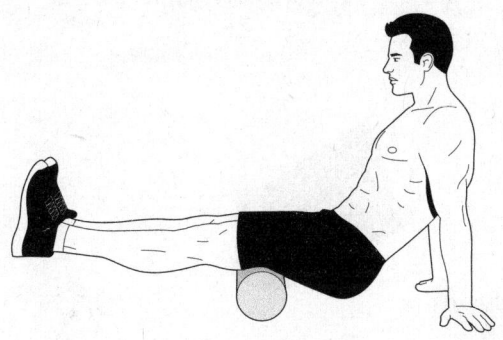

FOAM ROLL GROIN

Lie face down on the floor. Place a foam roller parallel to your body. Put your elbows on the floor for support. Position your right thigh nearly perpendicular to your body, with the inner portion of your thigh just above the level of your knee, resting on top of the roller. Roll your body toward the right until the roller reaches your pelvis. Then roll back and forth. Repeat with the roller on your left thigh.

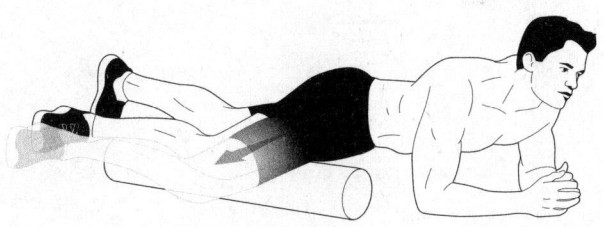

FOAM ROLL THORACIC SPINE

Lie face up with a foam roller under your upper back, at the tops of your shoulder blades. Cross your arms over your chest or clasp behind your head with elbows back. Your knees should be bent, with your feet flat on the floor. Raise your hips so they're slightly elevated off the floor. Roll back and forth over your shoulder blades and your mid- and upper back.

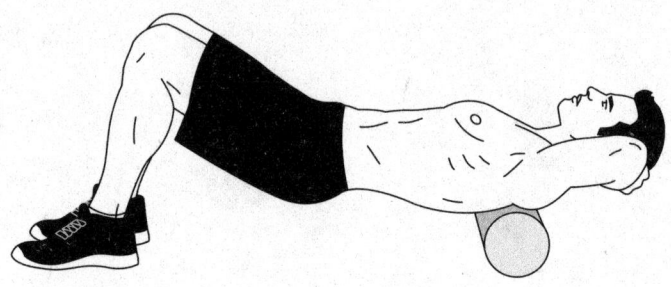

FOAM ROLL LUMBAR SPINE

Lie face up with a foam roller under your midback, knees bent and feet flat on the floor. Place your hands on the floor for support. Raise your hips slightly and roll until the roller reaches the top of your glutes. Roll back and forth over your lower back.

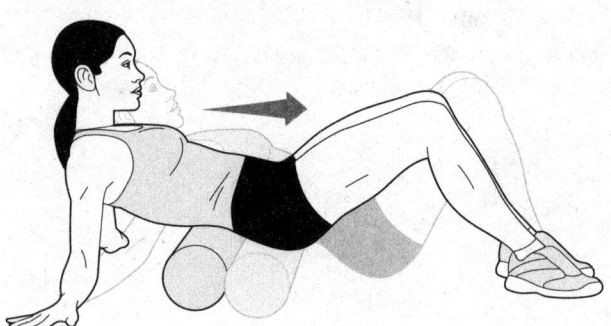

ACKNOWLEDGMENTS

This book is a product of decades of pushing myself to succeed while simultaneously encouraging others to push for success as well.

Although the concept of fitness motivation is simple, the task of taking this amorphous subject and creating evidence-based scientific clarity proved much more difficult. *Push* is the product of five years of writing, research, and revision, made possible by a collaborative effort with my friend and writing partner Mike Zimmerman. I am always grateful for his wisdom and guidance.

I am thankful to my agent, David Black, and editor, Michele Eniclerico, both of whom have championed my progress and encouraged me to continue through countless edits. I could not have gotten this across the finish line without their support.

I would not understand the concept of pushing myself without the tens of thousands of patients who I have been fortunate enough to care for over the years at Hospital for Special Surgery. Playing in a soccer game, running a marathon, climbing a mountain, doing a triathlon, each patient that I care for has a unique goal. When one of my patients meets their goal, and when I am fortunate enough to help along the way, I learn. With that knowledge, I am better able to help my other patients succeed. Thank you for entrusting me to care for your aches and pains while simultaneously helping you pursue your dreams.

I am equally thankful for the tens of thousands of people who have joined our IronStrength fitness community programs over the years. Our community is a mix of people from all walks of life, all ages, shapes, and sizes. The commonality is that everyone wants to move and be healthy. By learning how to encourage so many different people to push their bodies and minds, I developed a better understanding of how to harness and prescribe fitness motivation.

Finally, I want to acknowledge my incredible colleagues at Hospital for Special Surgery, friends, and family, all of whom have been incredibly supportive over months and years. I would not be who I am today without their support and encouragement.

NOTES

Introduction

1. C. G. Abildso, S. M. Daily, M. R. Umstattd Meyer, C. K. Perry, and A. Eyler, "Prevalence of Meeting Aerobic, Muscle-Strengthening, and Combined Physical Activity Guidelines During Leisure Time Among Adults, by Rural-Urban Classification and Region—United States, 2020," *Morbidity and Mortality Weekly Report* 72 (2023): 85–89, http://dx.doi.org/10.15585/mmwr.mm7204a1.
2. Centers for Disease Control and Prevention, "Adult Physical Inactivity Outside of Work," January 31, 2025, https://www.cdc.gov/physicalactivity/data/inactivity-prevalence-maps/index.html.
3. Armin Garmany, Satsuki Yamada, and Andre Terzic, "Longevity Leap: Mind the Healthspan Gap," *npj Regenerative Medicine* 6 (2021), art. no. 57, https://doi.org/10.1038/s41536-021-00169-5.
4. Armin Garmany, Satsuki Yamada, and Andre Terzic, "Global Healthspan-Lifespan Gaps Among 183 World Health Organization Member States," *JAMA Network Open* 7, no. 12 (2024): e2450241, https://doi.org/10.1001/jamanetworkopen.2024.50241.
5. A. Leroux, E. Cui, E. Smirnova, J. Muschelli, J. A. Schrack, and C. M. Crainiceanu, "NHANES 2011-2014: Objective Physical Activity Is the Strongest Predictor of All-Cause Mortality," *Medicine and Science in Sports and Exercise* 56, no. 10 (October 1, 2024): 1926–34, https://doi.org/10.1249/MSS.0000000000003497.

Chapter 1: What Is Movement?

1. World Health Organization, "Physical Activity," fact sheet, June 26, 2024, https://www.who.int/news-room/fact-sheets/detail/physical-activity; Dong Hoon Lee, Leandro F. M. Rezende, Hee-Kyung Joh, et al., "Long-Term Leisure-Time Physical Activity Intensity and All-Cause and Cause-

Specific Mortality: A Prospective Cohort of US Adults," *Circulation* 26, no. 7 (2022): 523–34, https://doi.org/10.1161/CIRCULATIONAHA .121.058162; J. P. Kirwan, J. Sacks, and S. Nieuwoudt, "The Essential Role of Exercise in the Management of Type 2 Diabetes," *Cleveland Clinic Journal of Medicine* 84, no. 7, suppl. 1 (July 2017): S15–S21, https://doi .org/10.3949/ccjm.84.s1.03; E. Stamatakis, M. N. Ahmadi, C. M. Frie-denreich, et al., "Vigorous Intermittent Lifestyle Physical Activity and Cancer Incidence Among Nonexercising Adults: The UK Biobank Ac-celerometry Study," *JAMA Oncology* 9, no. 9 (2023): 1255–59, https:// doi.org/10.1001/jamaoncol.2023.1830.

2. U. Ekelund, H. A. Ward, T. Norat, et al., "Physical Activity and All-Cause Mortality Across Levels of Overall and Abdominal Adiposity in European Men and Women: The European Prospective Investigation into Cancer and Nutrition Study (EPIC)," *American Journal of Clinical Nutrition* 101, no. 3 (2015): 613–21, https://doi.org/10.3945/ajcn.114 .100065.

3. J. J. Edwards, A. H. P. Deenmamode, M. Griffiths, et al., "Exercise Train-ing and Resting Blood Pressure: A Large-Scale Pairwise and Network Meta-Analysis of Randomised Controlled Trials," *British Journal of Sports Medicine* 57, no. 20 (October 2023): 1317–26, https://doi.org/10.1136 /bjsports-2022-106503.

4. B. C. Lee and J. Lee, "Cellular and Molecular Players in Adipose Tissue Inflammation in the Development of Obesity-Induced Insulin Resis-tance," *Biochimica et Biophysica Acta* 1842, no. 3 (2014): 446–62, https:// doi.org/10.1016/j.bbadis.2013.05.017; M. Blüher, "Adipose Tissue In-flammation: A Cause or Consequence of Obesity-Related Insulin Resis-tance?," *Clinical Science* 130, no. 18 (2016): 1603–14, https://doi.org/10 .1042/CS20160005.

5. S. Dimitrov, E. Hulteng, and S. Hong, "Inflammation and Exercise: In-hibition of Monocytic Intracellular TNF Production by Acute Exercise via ß-Adrenergic Activation," *Brain, Behavior, and Immunity* 61 (2017): 60–68, https://doi.org/10.1016/j.bbi.2016.12.017.

6. Érica Cerqueira, Daniel A. Marinho, Henrique P. Neiva, and Olga Lou-renço, "Inflammatory Effects of High and Moderate Intensity Exercise— A Systematic Review," *Frontiers in Physiology* 10 (2020): 550, https://doi .org/10.3389/fphys.2019.01550.

7. M. C. K. Severinsen and B. K. Pedersen, "Muscle-Organ Crosstalk: The Emerging Roles of Myokines," *Endocrine Reviews* 41, no. 4 (August 1, 2020): 594–609, https://doi.org/10.1210/endrev/bnaa016; erratum in *Endocrine Reviews* 42, no. 1 (January 28, 2021): 97–99, https://doi.org /10.1210/endrev/bnaa024.

8. Ceereena Ubaida-Mohien, Marta Gonzalez-Freire, Alexey Lyashkov, et al., "Physical Activity Associated Proteomics of Skeletal Muscle: Being Physically Active in Daily Life May Protect Skeletal Muscle from Aging," *Frontiers in Physiology* 10 (2019): 312, https://doi.org/10.3389/fphys.2019.00312.

9. T. Lohman, G. Bains, S. Cole, L. Gharibvand, L. Berk, and E. Lohman, "High-Intensity Interval Training Reduces Transcriptomic Age: A Randomized Controlled Trial," *Aging Cell* 22 (2023): e013841, https://doi.org/10.1111/acel.13841.

10. A. C. Letsinger, J. Z. Granados, S. E. Little, and J. T. Lightfoot, "Alleles Associated with Physical Activity Levels Are Estimated to Be Older Than Anatomically Modern Humans," *PLOS One* 14, no. 4 (2019): e0216155, https://doi.org/10.1371/journal.pone.0216155.

11. MoTrPAC Study Group, Lead Analysts, "Temporal Dynamics of the Multi-omic Response to Endurance Exercise Training," *Nature* 629 (2024): 174–83, https://doi.org/10.1038/s41586-023-06877-w; N. G. Vetr, N. R. Gay, MoTrPAC Study Group, et al., "The Impact of Exercise on Gene Regulation in Association with Complex Trait Genetics," *Nature Communications* 15, no. 3346 (2024), https://doi.org/10.1038/s41467-024-45966-w.

12. Larry A. Tucker, "Physical Activity and Telomere Length in U.S. Men and Women: An NHANES Investigation," *Preventive Medicine* 100 (2017): 145–51, https://doi.org/10.1016/j.ypmed.2017.04.027.

13. U.S. Department of Health and Human Services, *Physical Activity Guidelines for Americans,* 2nd ed. (U.S. Department of Health and Human Services, 2018), https://health.gov/sites/default/files/2019-09/Physical_Activity_Guidelines_2nd_edition.pdf.

14. E. Stamatakis, M. N. Ahmadi, J. M. R. Gill, et al., "Association of Wearable Device-Measured Vigorous Intermittent Lifestyle Physical Activity with Mortality," *Nature Medicine* 28 (2022): 2521–29, https://doi.org/10.1038/s41591-022-02100-x.

15. M. N. Ahmadi, P. J. Clare, P. T. Katzmarzyk, Borja Del Pozo Cruz, I. Min Lee, and Emmanuel Stamatakis, "Vigorous Physical Activity, Incident Heart Disease, and Cancer: How Little Is Enough?," *European Heart Journal* 43, no. 46 (December 7, 2022): 4801–14, https://pubmed.ncbi.nlm.nih.gov/36302460/.

16. Anthony Wolfe, Heath Burton, Emre Vardarli, and Edward Coyle, "Hourly 4-s Sprints Prevent Impairment of Postprandial Fat Metabolism from Inactivity," *Medicine and Science in Sports and Exercise* 52, no. 10 (October 2020): 2262–69, https://doi.org/10.1249/MSS.0000000000002367.

Chapter 2: Push Yourself

1. A. E. Bauman, M. Kamada, R. S. Reis, et al., "An Evidence-Based Assessment of the Impact of the Olympic Games on Population Levels of Physical Activity," *Lancet* 31, no. 398 (July 31, 2021): 456–64, https://doi.org/10.1016/S0140-6736(21)01165-X.

2. A. R. Sutin, Y. Stephan, M. Luchetti, et al., "Differential Personality Change Earlier and Later in the Coronavirus Pandemic in a Longitudinal Sample of Adults in the United States," *PLOS One* 17, no. 9 (2022): e0274542, https://doi.org/10.1371/journal.pone.0274542.

3. Zachary J. Ward, Sara N. Bleich, Angie L. Cradock, et al., "Projected U.S. State-Level Prevalence of Adult Obesity and Severe Obesity," *New England Journal of Medicine* 381 (2019): 2440–50, https://doi.org/10.1056/NEJMsa1909301.

4. American Diabetes Association, "Statistics about Diabetes," accessed March 31, 2025, https://www.diabetes.org/about-us/statistics/about-diabetes.

5. Joana Araujo, Jianwen Cai, and June Stevens, "Prevalence of Optimal Metabolic Health in American Adults: National Health and Nutrition Examination Survey 2009–2016," *Metabolic Syndrome and Related Disorders* 17, no. 1 (2019): 46–52, https://doi.org/10.1089/met.2018.0105.

6. Aaron Yao, Shengyu Zhou, Joyce Cheng, and Dae Hyun Kim, "Self-Reported Frailty and Health Care Utilization in Community-Dwelling Middle-Aged and Older Adults in the United States," *Journal of the American Medical Directors Association* 24, no. 4 (2022): 517–18, https://doi.org/10.1016/j.jamda.2022.12.007.

7. MedLine Plus, "Is Longevity Determined by Genetics?," accessed April 1, 2025, https://medlineplus.gov/genetics/understanding/traits/longevity/.

8. National Academy of Medicine, "Social Determinants of Health 101 for Health Care: Five plus Five," NAM Perspectives, 2017, https://nam.edu/social-determinants-of-health-101-for-health-care-five-plus-five.

9. National Academy of Medicine, "Social Determinants of Health 101."

Chapter 3: Motivation Is a Big Word

1. A. Baillot, S. Chenail, N. Barros Polita, et al., "Physical Activity Motives, Barriers, and Preferences in People with Obesity: A Systematic Review," *PLOS One* 16, no. 6 (2021): e0253114, https://doi.org/10.1371/journal.pone.0253114.

2. Richard Ryan and Edward Deci, "Self-Determination Theory and the Facilitation of Intrinsic Motivation, Social Development, and Well-

Being," *American Psychologist* 55, no. 1 (January 2000): 68–78, https://doi
.org/10.1037110003-066X.55.1.68.

3. S. Aral and C. Nicolaides, "Exercise Contagion in a Global Social Network," *Nature Communications* 8 (2017): 14753, https://doi.org/10.1038
/ncomms14753.

4. M. J. Biondolillo and D. B. Pillemer, "Using Memories to Motivate Future Behavior: An Experimental Exercise Intervention," *Memory* 23, no.
3 (2015): 390–402, https://doi.org/10.1080/09658211.2014.889709.

5. Cyrielle Billon, Emmalie Schoepke, Amer Avdagic, et al., "A Synthetic
ERR Agonist Alleviates Metabolic Syndrome," *Journal of Pharmacology
and Experimental Therapeutics* 388, no. 2 (September 23, 2023): 232–40,
https://doi.org/10.1124/jpet.123.001733.

6. Ronnie Blazev, Christian S. Carl, Yaan-Kit Ng, et al., "Phosphopro-
teomics of Three Exercise Modalities Identifies Canonical Signaling and
C18ORF25 as an AMPK Substrate Regulating Skeletal Muscle Function," *Cell Metabolism* 34, no. 10 (2022): 1561–77, https://doi.org/10
.1016/j.cmet.2022.07.003.

7. X. Qabrati, I. Kim, A. Ghosh, et al., "Transgene-Free Direct Conversion
of Murine Fibroblasts into Functional Muscle Stem Cells," *npj Regenerative Medicine* 8 (August 8, 2023): 43, https://doi.org/10.1038/s41536
-023-00317-z.

Chapter 4: Rescuing Your Motivation from Bad Influences

1. Rachel L. Ruttan and Loran F. Nordgren, "The Strength to Face the
Facts: Self-Regulation Defends Against Defensive Information Processing," *Organizational Behavior and Human Decision Processes* 137 (2016): 86–
98, https://doi.org/10.1016/j.obhdp.2016.06.006.

2. N. Bevan, K. S. O'Brien, C. Y. Lin, et al., "The Relationship Between
Weight Stigma, Physical Appearance Concerns, and Enjoyment and Tendency to Avoid Physical Activity and Sport," *International Journal of Environmental Research and Public Health* 18, no. 19 (September 22, 2021):
9957, https://doi.org/10.3390/ijerph18199957.

3. K. L. Olson, S. P. Goldstein, R. R. Wing, D. M. Williams, K. E. Demos,
and J. L. Unick, "Internalized Weight Bias Is Associated with Perceived
Exertion and Affect During Exercise in a Sample with Higher Body
Weight," *Obesity Science and Practice* 7, no. 4 (April 6, 2021): 405–14,
https://doi.org/10.1002/osp4.494.

4. Boris Cheval, Eda Tipura, Nicolas Burra, et al., "Avoiding Sedentary
Behaviors Requires More Cortical Resources Than Avoiding Physical
Activity: An EEG Study," *Neuropsychologia* 119 (2018): 68–80, https://doi
.org/10.1016/j.neuropsychologia.2018.07.029.

5. T. McElroy, D. L. Dickinson, N. Stroh, and C. A. Dickinson, "The Physical Sacrifice of Thinking: Investigating the Relationship Between Thinking and Physical Activity in Everyday Life," *Journal of Health Psychology* 21, no. 8 (2016): 1750–57, https://doi.org/10.1177/1359105314565827.

6. Global Wellness Institute, "2018 Global Wellness Economy Monitor," report, 2018, https://globalwellnessinstitute.org/industry-research/2018-global-wellness-economy-monitor/.

7. BlueCross BlueShield, "The Health of Millennials," report, 2019, https://www.bcbs.com/news-and-insights/report/the-health-of-millennials.

8. S. H. Woolf and H. Schoomaker, "Life Expectancy and Mortality Rates in the United States, 1959–2017," *JAMA* 322, no. 2 (2019): 1996–2016, https://doi.org/10.1001/jama.2019.16932.

9. Grand View Research, "Dietary Supplements Market Size, Share and Trends Analysis Report by Ingredient (Vitamins, Minerals), by Form, by Application, by End User, by Distribution Channel, by Region, and Segment Forecasts, 2022–2030," report, 2024, https://www.grandviewresearch.com/industry-analysis/dietary-supplements-market-report.

10. Statista, "Revenue of the Fitness, Health and Gym Club Industry in the United States from 2012 to 2022," 2025, https://www.statista.com/statistics/605223/us-fitness-health-club-market-size-2007-2021/.

11. N. Hagura, P. Haggard, and J. Diedrichsen, "Perceptual Decisions Are Biased by the Cost to Act," *Elife,* February 21, 2017, 6, https://doi.org/10.7554/eLife.18422.

12. D. S. Teixeira, V. Bastos, A. J. Andrade, A. L. Palmeira, and P. Ekkekakis, "Individualized Pleasure-Oriented Exercise Sessions, Exercise Frequency, and Affective Outcomes: A Pragmatic Randomized Controlled Trial," *International Journal of Behavioral Nutrition and Physical Activity* 21, no. 1 (August 5, 2024): 85, https://doi.org/10.1186/s12966-024-01636-0.

13. K. L. Milkman, D. Gromet, H. Ho, et al., "Megastudies Improve the Impact of Applied Behavioral Science," *Nature* 600 (2021): 478–83, https://doi.org/10.1038/s41586-021-04128-4.

14. M. S. Patel, D. S. Small, J. D. Harrison, et al., "Effectiveness of Behaviorally Designed Gamification Interventions with Social Incentives for Increasing Physical Activity Among Overweight and Obese Adults Across the United States: The STEP UP Randomized Clinical Trial," *JAMA Internal Medicine* 179, no. 12 (2019): 1624–32, https://doi.org/10.1001/jamainternmed.2019.350.

15. Katherine L. Milkman, Julia A. Minson, and Kevin G. M. Volpp, "Holding the Hunger Games Hostage at the Gym: An Evaluation of Temptation Bundling," *Management Science* 60, no. 2 (2013): 283–99, https://doi.org/10.1287/mnsc.2013.1784.

16. Neel P. Chokshi, Srinath Adusumalli, Dylan S. Small, et al., "Loss-Framed Financial Incentives and Personalized Goal-Setting to Increase Physical Activity Among Ischemic Heart Disease Patients Using Wearable Devices: The ACTIVE REWARD Randomized Trial," *Journal of the American Heart Association* 7 (2018): e009173, https://doi.org/10.1161/JAHA.118.009173.

Chapter 5: Knowledge

1. M. Viswanathan, C. E. Golin, C. D. Jones, et al., "Interventions to Improve Adherence to Self-Administered Medications for Chronic Diseases in the United States: A Systematic Review," *Annals of Internal Medicine* 157, no. 11 (2012): 785–95, https://doi.org/10.7326/0003-4819-157-11-201212040-00538.

2. A. Akincigil, J. R. Bowblis, C. Levin, S. Jan, M. Patel, and S. Crystal, "Long-Term Adherence to Evidence Based Secondary Prevention Therapies After Acute Myocardial Infarction," *Journal of General Internal Medicine* 23, no. 2 (2008): 115–21, https://doi.org/10.1007/s11606-007-0351-9.

3. S. Zhu, D. Sinha, M. Kirk, et al., "Effectiveness of Behavioural Interventions with Motivational Interviewing on Physical Activity Outcomes in Adults: Systematic Review and Meta-analysis," *British Medical Journal* 386 (2024): e078713, https://doi.org10.1136/bmj-2023-078713.

4. Z. Song and K. Baicker, "Effect of a Workplace Wellness Program on Employee Health and Economic Outcomes: A Randomized Clinical Trial," *JAMA* 321, no. 15 (2019): 1491–1501, https://doi.org/10.1001/jama.2019.3307.

5. D. E. R. Warburton and S. S. D. Bredin, "Health Benefits of Physical Activity: A Systematic Review of Current Systematic Reviews," *Current Opinion in Cardiology* 32, no. 5 (2017): 541–56, https://doi.org/10.1097/HCO.0000000000000437.

6. J. A. Gibbons, S. A. Lee, and W. R. Walker, "The Fading Affect Bias Begins Within 12 Hours and Persists for 3 Months," *Applied Cognitive Psychology* 25 (2011): 663–72, https://doi.org/10.1002/acp.1738.

7. J. A. Litman, "Interest and Deprivation Factors of Epistemic Curiosity," *Personality and Individual Differences* 44 (2008): 1585–95, https://doi.org/10.1016/j.paid.2008.01.014.

8. C. Kidd and B. Y. Hayden, "The Psychology and Neuroscience of Curiosity," *Neuron* 88, no. 3 (November 4, 2015): 449–60, https://doi.org/10.1016/j.neuron.2015.09.010.

9. E. Isikman, D. J. MacInnis, G. Ülkümen, and L. A. Cavanaugh, "The Effects of Curiosity-Evoking Events on Activity Enjoyment," *Journal of*

Experimental Psychology: Applied 22, no. 3 (2016): 319–30, https://doi.org
/10.1037/xap0000089.

Chapter 6: Emotion

1. S. H. Woolf and H. Schoomaker, "Life Expectancy and Mortality Rates in the United States, 1959–2017," *JAMA* 322, no. 20 (2019): 1996–2016, https://doi.org/10.1001/jama.2019.16932.
2. Lunna Lopes, Ashley Kirzinger, Grace Sparks, Mellisha Stokes, and Mollyann Brodie, "KFF/CNN Mental Health In America Survey," KFF, report, October 5, 2022, https://www.kff.org/report-section/kff-cnn-mental-health-in-america-survey-findings/.
3. Aaron White, I-Jen P. Castle, Ralph Hingson, and Patricia Powell, "Using Death Certificates to Explore Changes in Alcohol-Related Mortality in the United States, 1999–2017," *Alcoholism: Clinical and Experimental Research* 44, no. 1 (January 2020): 178–87, https://doi.org/10.1111/acer.14239.
4. J. M. Twenge, A. B. Cooper, T. E. Joiner, M. E. Duffy, and S. G. Binau, "Age, Period, and Cohort Trends in Mood Disorder Indicators and Suicide-Related Outcomes in a Nationally Representative Dataset, 2005–2017," *Journal of Abnormal Psychology* 128, no. 3 (2019): 185–99, https://doi.org/10.1037/abn0000410.
5. A. Heissel, D. Heinen, L. L. Brokmeier, et al., "Exercise as Medicine for Depressive Symptoms? A Systematic Review and Meta-analysis with Meta-regression," *British Journal of Sports Medicine* 57, no. 16 (August 2023): 1049–57, https://bjsm.bmj.com/content/early/2023/02/14/bjsports-2022-106282.
6. S. Fallah-fini, A. Adam, L. J. Cheskin, S. M. Bartsch, and B. Y. Lee, "The Additional Costs and Health Effects of a Patient Having Overweight or Obesity: A Computational Model," *Obesity* (Silver Spring) 25, no. 10 (2017): 1809–15, https://doi.org/10.1002/oby.21965.
7. J. Zagorsky, "Wealth and Weight," chap. 26 in *Oxford Handbook of Economics and Human Biology,* ed. John Komlos and Inas R. Kelly, online ed. (Oxford University Press, 2015), https://doi.org/10.1093/oxfordhb/9780199389292.013.20.
8. M. S. Patel, D. A. Asch, R. Rosin, et al., "Framing Financial Incentives to Increase Physical Activity Among Overweight and Obese Adults: A Randomized, Controlled Trial," *Annals of Internal Medicine* 164, no. 6 (2016): 385–94, https://doi.org/10.7326/M15-1635.
9. E. C. Willroth, G. Young, M. Tamir, and I. B. Mauss, "Judging Emotions as Good or Bad: Individual Differences and Associations with Psycho-

logical Health," *Emotion* 23, no. 7 (2023): 1876–90, https://doi.org/10.1037/emo0001220.

10. B. Wienke and D. Jekauc, "A Qualitative Analysis of Emotional Facilitators in Exercise," *Frontiers in Psychology* 7 (August 29, 2016): 1296, https://doi.org/10.3389/fpsyg.2016.01296.

11. Elisabeth Schafer, Robert B. Schafer, Patricia M. Keith, and Jana Böse, "Self-Esteem and Fruit and Vegetable Intake in Women and Men," *Journal of Nutrition Education* 31, no. 3 (May 1999): 153–60, https://doi.org/10.1016/S0022-3182(99)70422-X.

12. D. S. Lee and B. M. Way, "Perceived Social Support and Chronic Inflammation: The Moderating Role of Self-Esteem," *Health Psychology* 38, no. 6 (2019): 563–66, https://doi.org/10.1037/hea0000746.

13. Bas Verplanken and Jie Sui, "Habit and Identity: Behavioral, Cognitive, Affective, and Motivational Facets of an Integrated Self," *Frontiers in Psychology* 10 (July 9, 2019), https://doi.org/10.3389/fpsyg.2019.01504.

14. Felipe Caamaño-Navarrete, Pedro Ángel Latorre-Román, Iris Paola Guzmán-Guzmán, Juan Párraga Montilla, Daniel Jerez-Mayorga, and Pedro Delgado-Floody, "Lifestyle Mediates the Relationship Between Self-Esteem and Health-Related Quality of Life in Chilean Schoolchildren," *Psychology, Health, & Medicine* 27, no. 3 (2022): 638–48, https://doi.org/10.1080/13548506.2021.1934496.

15. L. Korn, E. Gonen, Y. Shaked, and M. Golan, "Health Perceptions, Self and Body Image, Physical Activity and Nutrition Among Undergraduate Students in Israel," *PLOS One* 8, no. 3 (2013): e58543, https://doi.org/10.1371/journal.pone.0058543.

Chapter 7: Belief

1. Albert Bandura, "Self-Efficacy: Toward a Unifying Theory of Behavioral Change," *Psychological Review* 84, no. 2 (1977): 191–215, https://doi.org/10.1037/0033-295x.84.2.191.

2. Albert Bandura, ed., *Self-Efficacy in Changing Societies* (Cambridge University Press, 1995).

3. E. Ouweneel, W. B. Schaufeli, and P. M. Le Blanc, "Believe, and You Will Achieve: Changes over Time in Self-Efficacy, Engagement, and Performance," *Applied Psychology: Health and Well-Being* 5, no. 2 (2013): 225–47, https://doi.org/10.1111/aphw.12008; Dale H. Schunk, "Self-Efficacy, Motivation, and Performance," *Journal of Applied Sport Psychology* 7, no. 2 (1995): 112–37, https://doiorg/10.1080/10413209508406961.

4. S. Meyler, L. Bottoms, and D. Muniz-Pumares, "Biological and Methodological Factors Affecting Response Variability to Endurance Training

and the Influence of Exercise Intensity Prescription," *Experimental Physiology* 106, no. 7 (2021): 1410–24, https://doi.org/10.1113/ep089565.

Chapter 8: Community

1. Albert Bandura, "Self-Efficacy: Toward a Unifying Theory of Behavioral Change," *Psychological Review* 84, no. 2 (1977): 191–215, https://doi.org/10.1037/0033-295x.84.2.191.

2. J. H. Fowler and N. A. Christakis, "Dynamic Spread of Happiness in a Large Social Network: Longitudinal Analysis over 20 Years in the Framingham Heart Study," *British Medical Journal* 337 (2008): a2338, https://doi.org/10.1136/bmj.a2338.

3. J. Holt-Lunstad, T. B. Smith, and J. B. Layton, "Social Relationships and Mortality Risk: A Meta-analytic Review," *PLOS Medicine* 7, no. 7 (2010): e1000316, https://doi.org/10.1371/journal.pmed.1000316.

4. David S. Lee and Baldwin M. Way, "Perceived Social Support and Chronic Inflammation: The Moderating Role of Self-Esteem," *Health Psychology* 38, no. 6 (2019): 563–66, https://doi.org/10.1037/hea0000746.

5. Y. C. Yang, C. Boen, K. Gerken, T. Li, K. Schorpp, and K. M. Harris, "Social Relationships and Physiological Determinants of Longevity Across the Human Life Span," *Proceedings of the National Academy of Sciences* 113, no. 3 (2016): 578–83, https://doi.org/10.1073/pnas.1511085112.

6. Virginia Thomas and Margarita Azmitia, "Motivation Matters: Development and Validation of the Motivation for Solitude Scale—Short Form (MSS-SF)," *Journal of Adolescence* 70 (2019): 33–42, https://doi.org/10.1016/j.adolescence.2018.11.004.

7. *Our Epidemic of Loneliness and Isolation: The U.S. Surgeon General's Advisory on the Healing Effects of Social Connection and Community* (U.S. Department of Health and Human Services, 2023), https://www.hhs.gov/sites/default/files/surgeon-general-social-connection-advisory.pdf.

8. F. Galkin, K. Kochetov, D. Koldasbayeva, et al., "Psychological Factors Substantially Contribute to Biological Aging: Evidence from the Aging Rate in Chinese Older Adults," *Aging* (Albany, N.Y.) 14, no. 18 (September 27, 2022): 7206–22, https://doi.org/10.18632/aging.204264.

Chapter 9: Preparing for the Push

1. M. B. Ruby, E. W. Dunn, A. Perrino, R. Gillis, and S. Viel, "The Invisible Benefits of Exercise," *Health Psychology* 30, no. 1 (January 2011): 67–74, https://doi.org/10.1037/a0021859.

2. D. Ekers, L. Webster, A. Van Straten, P. Cuijpers, D. Richards, and S. Gilbody, "Behavioural Activation for Depression: An Update of Meta-

analysis of Effectiveness and Subgroup Analysis," *PLOS One* 9, no. 6 (2014): e100100, https://doi.org/10.1371/journal.pone.0100100.

3. C. Martínez-Vispo, Ú. Martínez, A. López-Durán, E. Fernández Del Río, and E. Becoña, "Effects of Behavioural Activation on Substance Use and Depression: A Systematic Review," *Substance Abuse Treatment, Prevention, and Policy* 13, no. 1 (2018): art. no. 36, https://doi.org/10.1186/s13011-018-0173-2.

4. J. J. Heisz, M. G. M. Tejada, E. M. Paolucci, and C. Muir, "Enjoyment for High-Intensity Interval Exercise Increases During the First Six Weeks of Training: Implications for Promoting Exercise Adherence in Sedentary Adults," *PLOS One* 11, no. 12 (2016): e0168534, https://doi.org/10.1371/journal.pone.0168534.

5. K. Malik, M. Ibrahim, A. Bernstein, et al., "Behavioral Activation as an 'Active Ingredient' of Interventions Addressing Depression and Anxiety Among Young People: A Systematic Review and Evidence Synthesis," *BMC Psychology* 9, no. 150 (2021), https://doi.org/10.1186/s40359-021-00655-x.

6. K. L. Szuhany and M. W. Otto, "Efficacy Evaluation of Exercise as an Augmentation Strategy to Brief Behavioral Activation Treatment for Depression: A Randomized Pilot Trial," *Cognitive Behaviour Therapy* 49, no. 3 (May 2020): 228–41, https://doi.org/10.1080/16506073.2019.1641145.

7. Szu-chi Huang, Liyin Jin, and Ying Zhang, "Step by Step: Sub-goals as a Source of Motivation," *Organizational Behavior and Human Decision Processes* 141 (July 2017): 1–15, https://doi.org/10.1016/j.obhdp.2017.05.001.

Chapter 10: Your Exercise Prescription

1. Linda R. Archila, William Bostad, Michael J. Joyner, and Martin J. Gibala, "Simple Bodyweight Training Improves Cardiorespiratory Fitness with Minimal Time Commitment: A Contemporary Application of the 5BX Approach," *International Journal of Exercise Science* 14, no. 3 (2021): 93–100, https://digitalcommons.wku.edu/ijes/vol14/iss3/2.

2. C. J. Coleman, D. J. McDonough, Z. C. Pope, et al., "Dose-Response Association of Aerobic and Muscle-Strengthening Physical Activity with Mortality: A National Cohort Study of 416,420 US Adults," *British Journal of Sports Medicine* 56 (2022): 1218–23, http://dx.doi.org/10.1136/bjsports-2022-105519.

3. Mike Zimmerman, "This Man Will Make You Rich," *Men's Health* magazine, May 1, 2013, https://www.menshealth.com/trending-news/a19545960/investment-tips/.

Chapter 11: The Best Exercises No One Can Put a Price Tag On

1. Erin Wayman, "Becoming Human: The Evolution of Walking Upright," *Smithsonian* magazine, August 2012, https://www.smithsonianmag.com/science-nature/becoming-human-the-evolution-of-walking-upright-13837658/.

2. Zimin Song, Li Wan, Wenxiu Wang, et al., "Daily Stair Climbing, Disease Susceptibility, and Risk of Atherosclerotic Cardiovascular Disease: A Prospective Cohort Study," *Atherosclerosis* 386 (September 15, 2023), https://doi.org/10.1016/j.atherosclerosis.2023.117300.

3. N. A. Stens, E. A. Bakker, A. Mañas Bote, et al., "Relationship of Daily Step Counts to All-Cause Mortality and Cardiovascular Events," *Journal of the American College of Cardiology* 82, no. 15 (October 10, 2023): 1483–94, https://doi.org/10.1016/j.jacc.2023.07.029.

4. A. E. Paluch, S. Bajpai, D. R. Bassett, et al., "Daily Steps and All-Cause Mortality: A Meta-analysis of 15 International Cohorts," *Lancet Public Health* 7, no. 3 (March 2022): e219–e228, https://doi.org/10.1016/S2468-2667(21)00302-9.

5. Ian J. Wallace, Steven Worthington, David T. Felson, et al., "Knee Osteoarthritis Has Doubled in Prevalence Since the Mid-20th Century," *Proceedings of the National Academy of Sciences* 114, no. 35 (August 2017): 9332–36, https://doi.org/10.1073/pnas.1703856114.

6. J. Yang, C. A. Christophi, A. Farioli, et al., "Association Between Push-up Exercise Capacity and Future Cardiovascular Events Among Active Adult Men," *JAMA Network Open* 2, no. 2 (2019): e188341, https://doi.org/10.1001/jamanetworkopen.2018.8341.

7. S. Li, S. A. Lear, S. Rangarajan, et al., "Association of Sitting Time with Mortality and Cardiovascular Events in High-Income, Middle-Income, and Low-Income Countries," *JAMA Cardiology* 7, no. 8 (August 1, 2022): 796–807, https://doi.org/10.1001/jamacardio.2022.1581.

8. C. G. Araujo, C. G. de Souza e Silva, J. A. Laukkanen, et al., "Successful 10-Second One-Legged Stance Performance Predicts Survival in Middle-Aged and Older Individuals," *British Journal of Sports Medicine* 56 (2022): 975–80, http://dx.doi.org/10.1136/bjsports-2021-105360.

Chapter 13: Weeks 1 Through 4

1. David Dam, Davide Melcangi, Laura Pilossoph, and Aidan Toner-Rodgers, "What Have Workers Done with the Time Freed Up by Commuting Less?," Federal Reserve Bank of New York Liberty Street Economics, Oc-

tober 18, 2022, https://libertystreeteconomics.newyorkfed.org/2022/10/what-have-workers-done-with-the-time-freed-up-by-commuting-less/.

2. R. Sturm and D. A. Cohen, "Free Time and Physical Activity Among Americans 15 Years or Older: Cross-sectional Analysis of the American Time Use Survey," *Preventing Chronic Disease* 16 (2019): 190017, https://doi.org/10.5888/pcd16.190017.

3. Charlotte Ling and Tina Rönn, "Epigenetics in Human Obesity and Type 2 Diabetes," *Cell Metabolism* 29, no. 5 (2019): 1028–44, https://doi.org/10.1016/j.cmet.2019.03.009.

4. P. C. Dempsey, A. V. Rowlands, T. Strain, et al., "Physical Activity Volume, Intensity and Incident Cardiovascular Disease," *European Heart Journal* 43, no. 46 (2022): 4789–4800, https://doi.org/10.1093/eurheartj/ehac613.

5. D. G. Blackmore, M. A. Schaumberg, M. Ziaei, et al., "Long-Term Improvement in Hippocampal-Dependent Learning Ability in Healthy, Aged Individuals Following High Intensity Interval Training," *Aging and Disease* 16, no. 3 (2025): 1732–54, https://doi.org/10.14336/AD.2024.0642.

6. Y. Sawada, H. Ichikawa, N. Ebine, et al., "Effects of High-Intensity Anaerobic Exercise on the Scavenging Activity of Various Reactive Oxygen Species and Free Radicals in Athletes," *Nutrients* 15, no. 1 (January 1, 2023): 222, https://doi.org/10.3390/nu15010222.

7. M. Ashwell, L. Mayhew, J. Richardson, and B. Rickayzen, "Waist-to-Height Ratio Is More Predictive of Years of Life Lost Than Body Mass Index," *PLOS One* 9, no. 9 (2014): e103483, https://doi.org/10.1371/journal.pone.0103483.

8. B. G. Toresdahl, J. D. Metzl, J. Kinderknecht, et al., "Training Patterns Associated with Injury in New York City Marathon Runners," *British Journal of Sports Medicine* 57 (2023): 146–52, http://dx.doi.org/10.1136/bjsports-2022-105670.

9. T. G. Cotter and M. Rinella, "Nonalcoholic Fatty Liver Disease 2020: The State of the Disease," *Gastroenterology* 158, no. 7 (May 2020): 1851–64, https://doi.org/10.1053/j.gastro.2020.01.052.

10. D. J. van der Windt, V. Sud, H. Zhang, A. Tsung, and H. Huang, "The Effects of Physical Exercise on Fatty Liver Disease," *Gene Expression* 18, no. 2 (May 18, 2018): 89–101, https://doi.org/10.3727/105221617X15124844266408.

11. Angelique G. Brellenthin and Duck-chui Lee, "Comparative Effects of Aerobic, Resistance, and Combined Exercise on Sleep," abstract 38, presented at the American Heart Association's Epidemiology, Prevention/Lifestyle and Cardiometabolic Health (EPI/Lifestyle) Sessions 2022 (AHA/EPI 2022), March 3, 2022.

Chapter 14: #10 on "the Big List"

1. Abeer Alabduljabbar, Lyan Almana, Alanoud Almansour, et al., "Assessment of Fear of Failure Among Medical Students at King Saud University," *Frontiers in Psychology* 13 (March 10, 2022), https://doi.org/10.3389/fpsyg.2022.794700.

Part Four: Build Your Own Workouts

1. J. A. Bennie, J. Shakespear-Druery, and K. De Cocker, "Muscle-Strengthening Exercise Epidemiology: A New Frontier in Chronic Disease Prevention," *Sports Medicine—Open* 6, no. 40 (2020), https://doi.org/10.1186/s40798-020-00271-w.

2. J. Steele, J. P. Fisher, J. Giessing, et al., "Long-Term Time-Course of Strength Adaptation to Minimal Dose Resistance Training Through Retrospective Longitudinal Growth Modeling," *Research Quarterly for Exercise and Sport* 94, no. 4 (May 19, 2022): 1–18, https://doi.org/10.1080/02701367.2022.2070592.

3. J. Gorzelitz, B. Trabert, H. A. Katki, et al., "Independent and Joint Associations of Weightlifting and Aerobic Activity with All-Cause, Cardiovascular Disease and Cancer Mortality in the Prostate, Lung, Colorectal and Ovarian Cancer Screening Trial," *British Journal of Sports Medicine* 56 (2022): 1277–83, http://dx.doi.org/10.1136/bjsports-2021-105315.

4. E. Baz-Valle, B. J. Schoenfeld, J. Torres-Unda, J. Santos-Concejero, and C. Balsalobre-Fernández, "The Effects of Exercise Variation in Muscle Thickness, Maximal Strength and Motivation in Resistance Trained Men," *PLOS One* 14, no. 12 (2019): e0226989, https://doi.org/10.1371/journal.pone.0226989.

5. J. Afonso, R. Ramirez-Campillo, J. Moscão, et al., "Strength Training Is as Effective as Stretching for Improving Range of Motion: A Systematic Review and Meta-analysis," Meta ArXiv preprint, January 2021, https://doi.org/10.31222/osf.io/2tdfm.

6. B. J. Schoenfeld, M. D. Peterson, D. Ogborn, B. Contreras, and G. T. Sonmez, "Effects of Low- vs. High-Load Resistance Training on Muscle Strength and Hypertrophy in Well-Trained Men," *Journal of Strength and Conditioning Research* 29, no. 10 (October 2015): 2954–63, https://doi.org/10.1519/JSC.0000000000000958.

INDEX

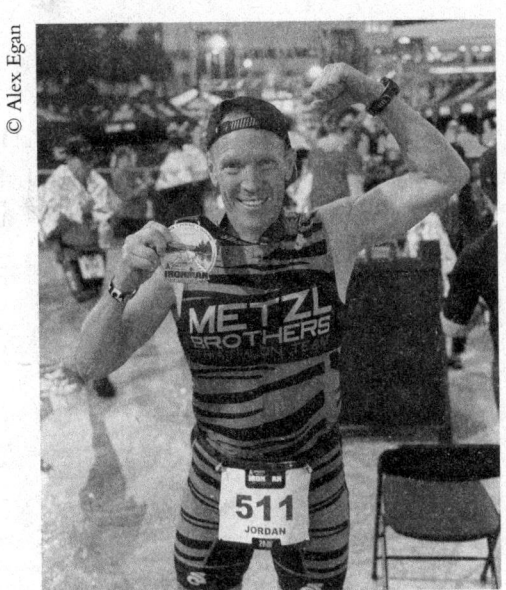

JORDAN D. METZL, MD (@DrJordanMetzl), is a prominent figure in the fields of sports medicine, orthopedics, fitness, and active longevity. Known for his expertise in treating sports injuries and promoting physical activity for preventive health, Dr. Metzl is not only a sports medicine physician but also an accomplished athlete and author. He is widely recognized for his ability to translate complex medical concepts into accessible, actionable advice for athletes and fitness enthusiasts of all levels.

As a clinician, Dr. Metzl serves as a sports medicine physician at Hospital for Special Surgery in New York City, where he provides comprehensive care for athletes of all ages and levels, from recreational enthusiasts to elite professionals. His approach to treatment emphasizes a combination of evidence-based medicine, cutting-edge therapies including regenerative medicine, and a deep understanding of the unique demands placed on the human body during physical activity.

He also recently started one of the first educational programs for medical students called "Prescribing the Medicine of Exercise," designed to teach physicians of the future how to prescribe exercise for preventive health. The seminar is held annually for second-year medical students at Weill Cornell Medical College, where he is on staff.

Beyond his clinical practice, Dr. Metzl is a passionate advocate for the importance of exercise in promoting overall health and well-being. He lectures at conferences, workshops, and public events, where he shares his insights on the benefits of physical activity and provides practical tips for injury prevention and rehabilitation. In 2010, he founded the IronStrength fitness community, one of the first physician-led fitness initiatives that provides free fitness classes for more than ten thousand people annually.

Dr. Metzl is also the author of *The Exercise Cure, The Athlete's Book of Home Remedies, Dr. Jordan Metzl's Workout Prescription,* and *Dr. Jordan Metzl's Running Strong,* all of which have earned acclaim for their blend of medical expertise, practical advice, and motivational insights. He has also partnered with *The New York Times* on a series of publications including "The 9 Minute Strength Workout" and "A User Manual for Your Knees."

In addition to his clinical practice and writing, Dr. Metzl is actively involved in research aimed at advancing our understanding of sports-related injuries and improving treatment outcomes. He is a sought-after media commentator, frequently appearing on television, on podcasts, and in print to share his expertise on topics related to sports medicine, fitness, and health.

He currently serves on the medical advisory board for the New York Road Runners club and has run forty marathons and fourteen Ironman triathlons.

Whether in the clinic, the classroom, or the media spotlight, he continues to inspire and empower others to achieve their fitness and health goals and live life to the fullest. He lives in New York City.

MIKE ZIMMERMAN is an award-winning health and fitness writer/editor with a body of work in magazines and books over twenty-five years. His work has appeared often in *Men's Health,* WebMD/Medscape, AARP, *The Wall Street Journal,* and many others. He was a 2022 National Magazine Award finalist and is the author of *The 14-Day Anti-Inflammatory Diet* and *Jet Lag Is for Suckers. Push* is his fourth collaboration with Dr. Metzl, including *The Athlete's Book of Home Remedies* and *Dr. Jordan Metzl's Workout Prescription.* Find him at zimwrites .com.

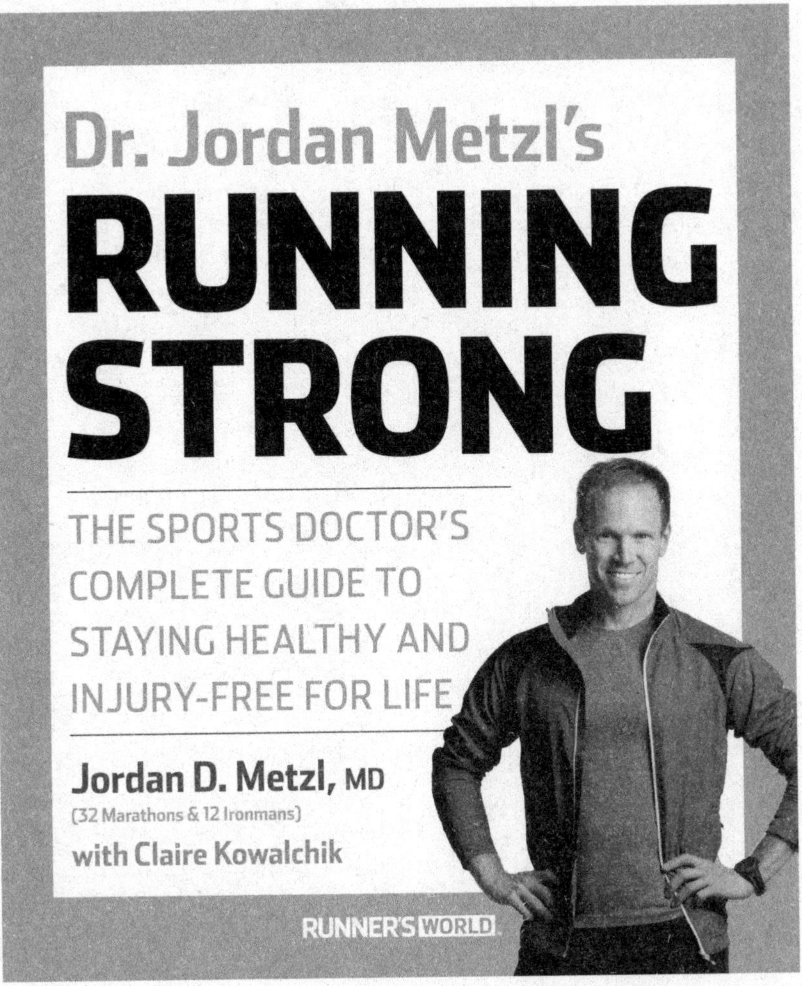

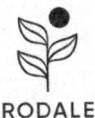